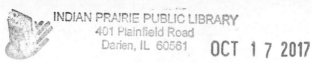

THE DIGESTIVE
HEALTH SOLUTION

Ben Brown is a naturopath, science writer and speaker. He teaches nutritional medicine, is on the advisory board at the UK College of Nutrition and Health (BCNH), speaks regularly at international conferences and workshops, and contributes to industry magazines and scientific journals. Ben also works in the research and development of nutraceuticals and has previously maintained a private practice.

THE DIGESTIVE HEALTH SOLUTION

Your personalized five-step plan for inside-out digestive wellness

BENJAMIN I. BROWN, ND

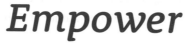

Empower

practical self-help tools by leading experts

First published 2015. This edition published 2017.

Exisle Publishing Pty Ltd
'Moonrising', Narone Creek Road, Wollombi,
NSW 2325, Australia
P.O. Box 60–490, Titirangi, Auckland 0642,
New Zealand
www.exislepublishing.com

A CiP record for this book is available from the National
Library of Australia.

ISBN 978-1-925335-38-5
Designed by Tracey Gibbs
Typeset in Miller Text
Cover illustration: VectorStock adapted by Tracey Gibbs

Printed in China

This book uses paper sourced under ISO 14001 guidelines
from well-managed forests and other controlled sources.

10 9 8 7 6 5 4 3 2 1

Disclaimer

This book is a general guide only and should never be a substitute for the skill, knowledge and experience of a qualified medical professional dealing with the facts, circumstances and symptoms of a particular case. The nutritional, medical and health information presented in this book is based on the research, training and professional experience of the author, and is true and complete to the best of their knowledge. However, this book is intended only as an informative guide; it is not intended to replace or countermand the advice given by the reader's personal physician. Because each person and situation is unique, the author and the publisher urge the reader to check with a qualified healthcare professional before using any procedure where there is a question as to its appropriateness. A physician should be consulted before beginning any exercise program. The author, publisher and their distributors are not responsible for any adverse effects or consequences resulting from the use of the information in this book. It is the responsibility of the reader to consult a physician or other qualified healthcare professional regarding their personal care. This book contains references to products that may not be available everywhere. The intent of the information provided is to be helpful; however, there is no guarantee of results associated with the information provided.

This book is for you, for asking questions, seeking answers and empowering yourself to improve your own health; we are all the authors of our own health and wellbeing.

And this book is also dedicated to the clinicians, educators and scientists who are selflessly championing a shift in medicine towards a more compassionate, natural and personalized approach, grounded in the connection to our food, lifestyle and environment.

CONTENTS

INTRODUCTION

I recently spoke at an international conference with the world-leading researcher and gastroenterologist Alessio Fasano, MD, who exclaimed, 'The microbiome, well I didn't see that coming!' And no one did. In the last few years ground-breaking discoveries have transformed the way we think about our digestive system. Ancient healing cultures have known for millenia that digestive health is the keystone of a healthy mind and body, and modern science has rediscovered the digestive health connection in ways that nobody would have dreamed possible just a decade ago.

The 'microbiome' Dr Fasano spoke of refers to the ecosystem of bacteria that lives in our digestive system, and only a decade ago we had no idea of its complexity and importance to our health. Thanks to huge advances in scientific research we now have a clearer picture. Today we know that the human digestive tract is home to a remarkable abundance of bacteria — at least tenfold more micro-organisms than cells that make up the human body — and that they influence not only our digestive health but the health of our whole body, including our immune system, cardiovascular system, metabolism, skin health and even our brain.

Disturbances in our gut bacteria have been linked to anxiety, depression, dementia, heart disease, allergies, autoimmune disease and weight gain, among many other illnesses. This is not to say it is the only cause, but it is an important part of the picture and helps us understand not only why these diseases occur, but how we could be better at treating them. The view that our overall health hangs so much on our digestive health is quite literally revolutionizing medicine. And, perhaps most importantly, we also have a better understanding of how we could influence our gut bacteria to improve our health and wellbeing and prevent illness before it even occurs, so there are important implications for wellness, healthy ageing and longevity, too.

So how do you know if your gut bacteria are out of balance? Digestive symptoms such as bloating, distension, pain, constipation and/or diarrhoea, discomfort and other niggling symptoms are strong indications. Research has shown that there are very robust correlations between these symptoms and the health of your gut bacteria. In general, if you have one or more of these symptoms regularly (which can be medically referred to as irritable bowel syndrome, or IBS) it is likely you are low in good bacteria, have more of the types linked to disease, and have lower overall diversity in your gut ecosystem. And just as low environmental diversity is an indicator of poor planetary health, low bacterial diversity in your gut is a signature of poor digestive health and ultimately bad news for the health of your whole body.

The good news is that scientists all over the world are working out why our digestive systems have become so unhealthy, and it has a lot to do with things we can do something about. It turns out that many of the things we have known are bad for us are probably bad for us because they are bad for our gut bacteria.

Modern diets, too much sugar, excess alcohol, environmental toxins, stress, lack of sleep, and too little exercise have all been linked to important changes in the microbiome. And the function of your body is also important: whether or not you have impaired digestion, inflammation in your digestive system, or your immune system is sensitive to certain foods, could all be important, for example. But there are also many other surprising reasons, and they are different for everyone.

The Digestive Health Solution is my modest answer for the millions of people who want to improve their digestive health and need a place to start. The internet, popular press and self-help books are awash with dubious information, but I have kept this book evidence-based so you know it is factual and really works. It is also highly personalized because there is no magic diet, drug or supplement. We are all unique, and therefore should have equally unique care.

A new view of health also permeates this book, the view that your body is a web of interconnected systems and that your health is dependent on your diet, lifestyle and environment. This may sound logical, but conventional medicine has for too long been concerned with dysfunction in one system (ignoring how digestive dysfunction could cause anxiety, for example) and with giving symptoms a name (such as IBS), then prescribing a corresponding drug (such as a pain medication); while this works well for acute, life-threatening illness it does not work well for chronic diet and lifestyle related disease, such as chronic digestive issues. This approach often fails to appreciate the underlying cause of the illness, the interconnection between systems and the role of nutritional and lifestyle changes as powerful therapeutic options that could eliminate your symptoms. The aim of this book is to emphasize these connections, explore why problems might occur and empower you with the tools you need to improve your health by addressing the underlying causes.

This second edition of *The Digestive Health Solution* has been updated to include important recent discoveries and is also shaped by the experiences of the thousands of people already using the book. Having given countless talks across many countries and spoken to hundreds of people using the book, I have learnt a lot from everyone and have distilled this into the new edition. You will find this an even better resource for helping transform your health and helping others do the same. After all, this book is for you.

PART 1

UNDERSTANDING DIGESTIVE TROUBLES

1

THE DIGESTIVE ILLNESS EPIDEMIC

Abdominal pain, bloating, discomfort and erratic bowel movements are the classic symptoms that define irritable bowel syndrome; however, symptoms of IBS are not just limited to your digestive system and can extend out to a host of related complaints ranging from muscle pain and fatigue to anxiety. If you suffer from these symptoms you are not alone. The number of people who suffer from these symptoms is extremely high and tends to range from at least 5 to 10 per cent of the general population, which makes IBS the most common gastrointestinal problem in the world.

For many years the symptoms of IBS have been dismissed as being 'all in the mind' (and were even historically named 'nervous colitis') or were linked to an unhealthy diet. However, we now know that both these assumptions are wrong, yet, even today, digestive complaints remain a source of great confusion. Subsequently, people who suffer from these symptoms also suffer from a great deal of frustration due to the lack of understanding about their illness.

Importantly, the conventional medical diagnosis of IBS is based only on a cluster of common symptoms, so by its very definition there are no functional causes. In other words, if you get labelled with IBS you have the symptoms but little attention is paid to what's actually going on in your digestive system to cause your discomfort. The lack of an objective diagnosis, such as a blood test, makes things even more challenging. And the complex nature of these digestive symptoms means that the disease frequently baffles not only the people who suffer from it but also health professionals who may misdiagnose or mismanage the disease.

There is no simple cure for the symptoms of IBS. Medications don't work very well for most people and none offer any hope of complete relief. Sadly, the most frequently used medications are painkillers or self-medication with dangerous narcotics, which provide modest symptom relief at best and are fraught with serious side effects. Perhaps not surprisingly, most people have been suffering for a very long time.

The majority of people affected with digestive complaints experience symptoms daily and for many years. A large survey of people with IBS revealed that 50 per cent had had symptoms for more than ten years and a remarkable 16 per cent had suffered for up to 30 years. Alarmingly, 57 per cent of people had symptoms daily, 25 per cent weekly, and 14 per cent monthly.[1] Living with a digestive illness can be life crippling.

The toll that digestive complaints can take on quality of life is frightening. Dietary restrictions, mood disturbances and symptoms such as pain, bloating, constipation and diarrhoea interfere profoundly with the ability to lead a normal life. On average, the symptoms of IBS restrict daily activities for about ten weeks out of each year, and can be so bad that when asked in a survey, people said that, given a choice, they would rather give up 25 per cent of their remaining life (an average of 15 years) than continue to live with their symptoms.[2]

The reason these symptoms remain a medical enigma is that underlying them is a complex process that is the result of multiple environmental factors influencing genetically susceptible people.[3] In other words, your digestive system is your weak spot and there could be a number of factors to blame for your symptoms. So, there is no single cause but rather multiple reasons why people develop poor gastrointestinal health. For this reason, identifying the cause is no simple task, and there is often more than one cause to blame.

Recent environmental and lifestyle changes help to explain why digestive complaints have become so common. It has been suggested that the symptoms of IBS, like other chronic diseases such as heart disease and obesity, are a disease of modern civilization. Indeed, as societies modernize, the prevalence of IBS becomes much higher.[4] With modernization comes dramatic lifestyle changes: increased psychological stress, sleep deprivation, dietary upheaval, decreased physical activity, social isolation, and exposure to drugs and pollutants — all typical features of modern life that can have adverse effects on digestive health.

Although a family history of IBS is not unusual and some genes have been identified that may increase susceptibility to digestive illness, it is generally accepted that genes only make a minor contribution to the disease. Rather, it is an array of environmental factors working in concert with a subtle genetic predisposition that is thought to be the underlying cause of IBS. In other words, for some people their gut is their weakness and this weakness may manifest as chronic, life-crippling symptoms given the right pressures.

While IBS continues to be dismissed as a set of symptoms with no known cause, this view has been seriously challenged by recent evidence that there are several clear causes of IBS that, when addressed, can result in significant improvement and even complete resolution of symptoms.

Further, the notion that IBS is not related to any underlying disturbance in the gastrointestinal system has also been proven to be wrong. Research has identified changes in the gastrointestinal system that help to explain many of the symptoms. The type of dysfunction may vary from person to person but there are commonalities that can nonetheless be identified with testing, and treated with remarkable results.

These discoveries offer a new view of poor digestive health as a complex problem that has tangible and very real underlying causes. This view also opens up the door for new hope because identifying and addressing the underlying cause of an illness is a powerful way to pave the road to recovery.

This book will take you on a journey through the latest research, helping you understand what is going on in your gut and why the health of your digestive system is linked to the health of your whole body. This book will also explore the reasons for your symptoms and empower you with the knowledge you need to get to the root cause of your illness, to reclaim your digestive health and total wellbeing.

NINE COMMON MEDICAL MYTHS ABOUT DIGESTIVE ILLNESS

Myth 1: It is all in your head

For a long time the symptoms of IBS have been thought to be purely psychological and people with chronic digestive complaints are sometimes still told that it's all in their head. Well, it *is* in your head, but not how you think! Several studies have found an increased incidence of stress, anxiety and even functional changes in the brains of people with IBS, but this is only half the picture.

Your head is part of your gastrointestinal system. This may sound like a crazy suggestion but your brain and gut are in constant communication via what is referred to scientifically as the gut–brain axis. The gut–brain axis is basically a network of nerves and hormones that closely link your digestive system and brain, sending messages so that your gut can tell your brain if you are hungry or full, and your brain can tell your gut if you are stressed or anxious. The interesting thing is that your gut can change your emotions, but more on that later.

So the truth is that your brain and gut are intimately interconnected, and dysfunction in one area can affect the other. Just as stress can cause digestive problems, digestive problems can cause stress. So if someone tells you it's all in your head, let them know politely that scientific research has proven that their brains are in their bowels. Stress, depression and anxiety are very common complaints in people suffering from digestive illness, but these afflictions are far more often a symptom rather than a cause.

Myth 2: There is no known cause

As you will find in this book, there are a lot of very different potential causes of your digestive complaints, and the symptoms are remarkably diverse, so understanding what's going on requires a big-picture view. This is why people with digestive complaints are frequently misdiagnosed and wrongly treated. Drug treatments for the symptoms of IBS rarely work well because of the narrow way they act.

The problem is that while a diagnosis (the classification of an illness based on symptoms or testing) can be useful, identifying the underlying cause is much more meaningful. Rather than being labelled with IBS, wouldn't you rather someone investigated every possible cause and helped you get to the reason for your symptoms?

The purpose of this book is to help you explore a wide range of possible causes of your symptoms and for you to achieve long-term relief by identifying and dealing with the reason for your problems in the first place, rather than being labelled with IBS and given little hope for recovery. Actually, there are many different reasons why people suffer from digestive symptoms and there is a lot you can do about it.

Myth 3: Your symptoms will go away with time

For some people, digestive troubles are intermittent and may even disappear with time but, unfortunately, most people constantly suffer and may have symptoms for the whole of their lives. Furthermore, there is evidence to suggest that having the symptoms of IBS increases your risk for Inflammatory Bowel Disease (IBD), a severe and crippling autoimmune condition. Some researchers believe that IBS is actually a mild precursor to IBD; in fact, the two diseases share many similarities and people with IBS are far more likely (up to fifteen times) to develop IBD.[5] Researchers also think that IBS may be linked to the development of conditions such as obesity, heart disease and type-2 diabetes because of poor digestion, nutrient absorption or changes in gut bacteria.[6]

The good news is that it is highly likely your symptoms will go away with time if you get to the underlying cause.

Putting up with symptoms in the hope that the condition will improve is not going to get you anywhere if you don't deal with the root cause of your problem. For example, if it turns out you have a food intolerance and something in your diet is aggravating your symptoms, you are unlikely to mysteriously get better with time, or with medication for that matter, if you keep eating the problem food.

While this book does not claim to be a miracle cure, it will empower you with the information and tools you need to take control of your health rather than live in the hope that things will just get better. If you do take action your symptoms may improve with time, and in some cases very fast.

Myth 4: Probiotic supplements are useless

The media loves an attention-grabbing headline and often misrepresents scientific research, and this is true for probiotic supplements. It's not that the people in the media are wrong or mischievous, it's that we need to be smarter when it comes to science reporting and believing media headlines.

When looking at the effect of dietary supplements like probiotics, it is important to review the research in its entirety. Unfortunately, isolated studies can be misleading and these are generally what are reported on. A headline might read 'Probiotic supplements are useless' but what do the thousands of other studies suggest?

Some probiotics have been shown to be tremendously effective for common digestive complaints such as bloating, pain and diarrhoea, but not all of them (even the ones that have shown some benefit) are effective for everybody. So the truth is, certain probiotics can be very helpful for some people. In fact, there is evidence to suggest that probiotics can not only relieve symptoms, they can also help improve the balance of your gut bacteria, which may well be a reason why people develop digestive problems in the first place.

Myth 5: Diet has nothing to do with it

Many people with digestive complaints identify diet as a trigger of their symptoms. Unfortunately, some dietary recommendations for IBS don't take into account newer research in this area and fall short of the mark by making simplistic, general healthy-eating guidelines that often don't help at all.

Following the popular recommendation to simply eat a healthy, balanced diet could spell disaster for a lot of people with digestive problems. There are many seemingly healthy foods that can aggravate symptoms and, although touted as being beneficial, may actually be the root cause of the problem.

As the old adage suggests, 'One person's food is another person's poison' and there really is no one-size-fits-all dietary approach. This book will help you identify common but perhaps surprising foods that may be a problem for you, and enable you to personalize your diet for optimal digestive health.

While dietary change is not the solution for everyone, for some people diet has everything to do with their symptoms. Diet *does* play a very important role when it comes to digestive illness, but perhaps not in the way you have been led to believe.

Myth 6: You need to eat more fibre

Early studies claimed that dietary fibre might be able to help people with symptoms such as bloating, pain, constipation or diarrhoea, and since then increasing fibre intake has been a popular recommendation. But these early studies had important flaws in the way they were conducted and we now know that for some people, fibre can make things a lot worse.

In fact, pioneering research into the dietary treatment of digestive illness has found that reducing specific dietary fibres can result in dramatic improvements in symptoms, which flies in the face of the 'eat more fibre' mantra. It also appears that the type of fibre you eat matters, with some able to aggravate symptoms while others can be used to provide relief.

So, if you have tried eating more fibre and found that it doesn't help much, or makes things worse, don't worry, you are not alone. Understanding how certain fibres can aggravate symptoms and why, as detailed in this book, will help you make dietary changes that don't send you into a symptom attack. You will also learn which types of fibre can really help get your digestive system back on track.

Myth 7: The symptoms are only in your gut

One of the biggest misunderstandings about digestive illness, and perhaps the human body in general, is that dysfunction in one area is not connected to another. Everything in the body is interconnected and works in synchrony. So ill health in the gut is linked to ill health throughout the rest of your body.

People with digestive problems commonly experience symptoms that affect their mental function, feelings, sleep, muscles, joints, pain sensitivity, physical energy, urination and sexual function. This is not due to random chance, it is because many of the disturbances in the gut are connected to, or are creating disturbances in, the rest of the body.

Instead of looking at your digestive symptoms as a problem affecting your gut, it is better to think of it as a complex issue that can affect many different areas of your body and result in an alarmingly wide range of symptoms beyond digestion.

Myth 8: Medications will fix the problem

Unfortunately, there are no medications that cure the symptoms of IBS and it is unlikely that a wonder drug will ever exist. There are some medications that are used to help control certain symptoms, such as severe diarrhoea, but the effectiveness of these for the most troubling symptoms, mainly abdominal pain and bloating, is disappointing.

The reason medications are unlikely to offer a cure for your digestive issues is that they have targeted effects, like on a cell receptor or biochemical pathway. For most people, their gut problems are the result of several widespread factors involving the gut, brain, immune and nervous systems, so a single medication is limited in addressing the wide variety of issues that are going on. And the symptoms themselves can be caused by a variety of different issues such as diet or changes in your gut bacteria. Logically then, identifying and dealing with the actual cause is going to be far more effective than treating the symptoms with a drug. Even if medications could and do provide relief, they may not be dealing with why the problem is there in the first place.

Myth 9: There is no cure

There is a cure for the various symptoms of IBS, but not in the traditional sense of a one-size-fits-all magic bullet. The cure varies from person to person and in most cases requires addressing multiple dietary, behavioural and lifestyle factors.

By addressing the personal and unique causes of your symptoms, you will be able to experience dramatic improvements in your symptoms and perhaps even cure your disease, but this will take some learning, personal exploration, trial and error and ongoing life-long preventative care.

This may seem like a lot to ask in today's quick-fix, pill-for-an-ill society, but the idea of an instant cure, as you already know, is often an illusion. Modern medicine does not have all the answers and it is important to understand that digestive illness can be a complex problem with many aggravating factors. You could ignore your symptoms and continue to suffer, or take your health into your own hands, adopt a proactive approach and enjoy the freedom of being symptom free.

2

DO YOU HAVE IBS?

Very simply, if you have abdominal pain, bloating, discomfort and erratic bowel movements, there is a good chance you have irritable bowel syndrome, or IBS. But there is a lot more to it than that, so let's look at IBS in more detail.

If you have the symptoms listed above, you are not alone. Up to one in five people suffer from IBS, making it the most common digestive problem that anyone experiences.[1] But despite how widespread the problem is, the medical diagnosis of IBS is grossly lacking and many people are misdiagnosed and sometimes incorrectly treated.[2] To make things worse, some medical professionals still hold on to the old and incorrect idea that it is all in people's heads, and dismiss the problem as a psychological disorder.

There is no single laboratory test that can identify whether or not you have IBS, so the way of identifying whether you have it is by using the Rome III Diagnostic Criteria for Functional Gastrointestinal Disorders. The Rome III criteria were developed to help assess various gastrointestinal problems by the Rome Foundation, a non-profit, independent expert committee who met in Rome, hence the name. The Rome III criteria is simply:

Recurrent abdominal pain or discomfort* at least three days a month over the last three months associated with two or more of the following:
1. Improvement with defecation.
2. Onset associated with a change in frequency of stool.
3. Onset associated with a change in form (appearance) of stool.

*Discomfort being an uncomfortable sensation and not pain.

In short, if you have occasional abdominal pain or discomfort and altered bowel movements over a period of at least three months, you have IBS. If you suffer from IBS I am sure you can quickly see that this is, well, a rather inadequate description, as the symptoms of IBS are in reality far more varied and often much more frequent. We will explore the symptoms in a lot more detail later.

The Rome III criteria also has three subtypes of IBS depending on whether you tend toward constipation, diarrhoea, or a combination of both:

Type 1: IBS with diarrhoea (IBS-D): Loose stools more than 25 per cent of the time and hard stools less than 25 per cent of the time.

Type 2: IBS with constipation (IBS-C): Hard stools more than 25 per cent of the time and loose stools less than 25 per cent of the time.

Type 3: IBS with mixed bowel habits or cyclic pattern (IBS-M): Both hard and soft stools more than 25 per cent of the time.

The problem with this classification is that many people will switch between each of these subtypes. Your predominant subtype may, however, be used to direct your treatment. For example, if you have IBS-D you might receive a drug to help stop the diarrhoea.

It is important to know that the Rome III criteria is more of an 'expert opinion' than it is based on the range of symptoms that people with IBS actually suffer from, and is more for research purposes than it is for working out if you actually have IBS. In fact, an expert review concluded that the accuracy of the Rome III criteria has not been established. In other words, it is not something you want to solely rely on.[3]

So what are the symptoms of IBS? Well, beyond the simple Rome III definitions there are a host of other symptoms that people with IBS are known to suffer from. Answer the following questionnaire to see if you are experiencing some of the more common symptoms.

THE IBS SYMPTOM QUESTIONNAIRE

Tick 'yes' if you typically have experienced these symptoms more than three days a week over the last month.

1. Do you suffer from abdominal pain or discomfort?

   No   Yes

2. Do you feel relief of pain or discomfort upon defecation?

   No   Yes

3. Does the pain or discomfort change with bowel movements?

   No   Yes

4. Do you feel bloated or distended?

   No   Yes

5. Do you have visible abdominal distention?

   No   Yes

6. Do you experience constipation (hard, pellet-like stools)?

   No   Yes

7. Do you experience diarrhoea (loose and runny stools)?

   No   Yes

8. Do you experience a combination of constipation and diarrhoea?

                                        No   Yes

9. Do you get abdominal pain and cramps?

                                        No   Yes

10. Do you suffer from excessive flatulence?

                                        No   Yes

11. Do you get a sense of urgency to rush to the bathroom?

                                        No   Yes

12. Do you strain upon defecation?

                                        No   Yes

13. Do you get more frequent stools at the onset of pain?

                                        No   Yes

14. Do you get looser stools at the onset of pain?

                                        No   Yes

15. Do you feel a sense of incomplete evacuation?

                                        No   Yes

16. Do you notice mucus in your stools?

                                        No   Yes

17. Do you experience reflux or heartburn?

                                        No   Yes

18. Are your symptoms worse after eating?

                                        No   Yes

19. Are your symptoms worse as the day progresses?

No   Yes

20. Are your symptoms related to stress?

No   Yes

21. Do you suffer from depression and/or anxiety?

No   Yes

22. Do you experience chronic fatigue and tiredness?

No   Yes

23. Do you suffer from muscle aches and pains?

No   Yes

If you answered 'yes' to questions 1, 2 or 3, you have IBS by the textbook definition. However, in reality there are a lot of other common symptoms and there is a good chance you have a lot more going on.

As you can see, there are many varied symptoms of IBS. Although you may not have all of these, you will have quite a few. It is important to understand that IBS is more than just the Rome III 'textbook' definition; it is actually a constellation of diverse symptoms ranging from digestive symptoms to problems that are not limited to your digestive system, such as chronic fatigue, anxiety or muscle pain.

UNDERSTANDING COMMON DIGESTIVE SYMPTOMS

Constipation

Constipation is very common; in fact, a large survey of over 10,000 people in the United States found that 14.7 per cent suffered from constipation and almost half of these people said they had been constipated for over five years.[4] Many of these people also met the criteria for IBS.

One of the difficulties with defining constipation is that no one seems to agree on what the definition is exactly. The opinion of medical professionals varies but one of the most popular is based on frequency, defining constipation as less than three bowel movements per week, although this is not a strictly accurate definition. And if you ask the average person what constipation is, they will tend not to focus on frequency at all and tell you constipation is related to symptoms such as straining, hard lumpy stools, bloating, abdominal discomfort, unproductive urges, inability to defecate at will, an excessive amount of time spent on the toilet or a feeling of incomplete evacuation.[5,6]

To further complicate things, what constitutes a 'normal' bowel movement seems to vary quite widely from person to person. When surveyed, most people (98 per cent) tend to report that they normally have between three bowel movements per day and three bowel movements per week. So you can see, a definition based solely on how frequently you move your bowels is not going to be very helpful.[7]

To help clarify things again, the Rome III criteria also has a definition of constipation:

Presence of two or more of the following symptoms over the last month:

1. straining during at least 25 per cent of defecations
2. lumpy or hard stools in at least 25 per cent of defecations
3. sensation of incomplete evacuation for at least 25 per cent of defecations
4. sensation of obstruction/blockage for at least 25 per cent of defecations
5. manual manoeuvres (that is, using your fingers, or pushing against your pelvic floor) to facilitate at least 25 per cent of defecations
6. fewer than three bowel movements per week.

Also, loose stools are rarely present without the use of laxatives.

You are forgiven if you lost interest after the word 'Presence'. Many people find this definition hard to grasp. Fortunately, a much easier to understand and perhaps more revealing definition of constipation was developed by a group from the University of Bristol in England which, incidentally, is known as the Bristol Stool Scale.[8] The great thing about the Bristol Stool Scale is that it is an easy visual reference guide that gives you an idea of whole-gut transit time, that is, the time it takes your food to pass from your mouth, through your digestive system and out the other end.

The average transit time is around 30 to 40 hours, with 70 hours (three days) at the upper range of normal.[9] Transit time in people with IBS may vary from just seven hours with diarrhoea, up to 96 hours with constipation.[10] A slow transit time based on the Bristol Stool Scale is an excellent indicator of constipation and is a more accurate indicator than how frequently you go.[11]

Simply, if you have a slow intestinal transit time you will have hard lumpy stools (Types 1 and 2 on the scale), which cause straining, difficulty and discomfort. Types 1 and 2 on the scale are a sign of constipation. If your stool is slow, it sits in your colon longer and tends to dry out because you reabsorb the water, hence the dry, compact shape.

Ideally your stools should be a Type 3, or even better a Type 4, which is soft and easy to pass. Higher numbers up the scale (5, 6 and 7) are the realm of rapid transit and watery diarrhoea.

The Bristol Stool Scale

Type 1 — Separate hard lumps like nuts (hard to pass)

Type 2 — Sausage shaped but lumpy

Type 3 — Like a sausage but with cracks on its surface

Type 4 — Like a sausage or snake, smooth and soft

Type 5 — Soft blobs with clear-cut edges (passed easily)

Type 6 — Fluffy pieces with ragged edges, a mushy stool

Type 7 — Watery, no solid pieces (entirely liquid)

Fast transit

Diarrhoea

Like constipation, diarrhoea is a surprisingly common problem in the general population. A survey of more than 1000 people in the United States found that as many as one in four people reported suffering from chronic diarrhoea.[12] It is estimated that about 70 per cent of people with IBS suffer from diarrhoea, and half of these people will have diarrhoea most of the time while the other half alternate between constipation and diarrhoea.[13]

Chronic diarrhoea is an incredibly stressful and troubling symptom to live with. Not knowing when you might have an episode, having to plan ahead and risking embarrassment, has a huge impact on a person's quality of life and psychological wellbeing and may cause fear, anxiety and panic. In fact, a survey at South Manchester University Hospital revealed that feelings of hopelessness because of the relentless and often poorly treated symptoms of IBS cause a lot of sufferers to go so far as contemplating suicide.[14]

And, in a vicious circle, stress and anxiety are known to decrease gut transit time and thus cause diarrhoea because your digestive system is under the control of your nervous system.[15] So in a catch-22, diarrhoea can cause stress that can trigger diarrhoea.

The general definition of IBS-related diarrhoea is loose (mushy) or watery stools more than 25 per cent of the time for at least three months. On the Bristol Stool Scale, diarrhoea would be a Type 6 or 7, indicating rapid transit.

If your diarrhoea is with every bowel motion, is watery, associated with excessive gas, weight loss and relatively recent (less than two weeks) you should seek immediate medical care as you can become severely dehydrated and need to be investigated for something more serious, like a parasitic infection or an underlying illness, that may be causing your symptoms.[16] In any case, if diarrhoea is your predominant symptom you should seek medical advice for the same reasons.

If you have had diarrhoea for a number of months and have been tested and nothing has been found, or it is intermittent with normal bowel movements, it is likely you have IBS. A number of experiments have found that people with IBS-related diarrhoea have subtle changes in gut function including increases in muscle contractions and a fast transit time.[17] This helps explain why diarrhoea may occur in IBS in the absence of common causes, and why after your tests come back negative you might be diagnosed with IBS.

It is also worth noting that another subtype of IBS called post-infectious IBS (PI-IBS) usually has diarrhoea as a predominant symptom.[18] As the name suggests, PI-IBS develops after gastrointestinal infection with a bacteria or parasite, such as traveller's diarrhoea. Sometimes infections like this can develop into IBS months or even years after the infectious organism is treated or your initial symptoms have passed.

Bloating

Abdominal bloating is one of the most troubling symptoms of IBS. In a survey where people with IBS were asked to rate their most bothersome symptoms, the vast majority said bloating was a far more significant symptom than physical pain.[19]

Bloating is when your abdomen feels distended, gassy, full, hard or tight and may also be visibly distended or swollen, though not always. The bloating associated with IBS has some unique characteristics. People with IBS who experience bloating frequently report:

- their abdomen is flat in the morning and worse in the evening
- it improves overnight
- it is better when lying down
- it is worse after eating
- it can be worse with stress
- it can occur quite quickly, in less than 10 minutes
- it is worse with constipation-predominant IBS (IBS-C)
- in women, it can be worse prior to menstruation.[20]

Feeling bloated and actually being distended or swollen are two different things. Although bloating is a common feature of IBS, only half of the people who feel bloated actually have a measurable increase in their abdomen, which if swollen can distend by up to 12 cm (4¾ in) in diameter.[21]

The reason for the differences between feeling bloated and being visually distended may be down to different underlying reasons for each unique symptom in the gut. Distention could be due to the excessive fermentation of fibre by gut bacteria, causing increased gas production and subsequent swelling,[22,23] while people with a particularly sensitive gut tend to feel bloated after eating because of the normal pressure from food on their gut wall, despite no measurable distention.[24]

If you find that your bloating or distention does not vary with the time of day or when eating, and it is constant and getting progressively worse, you should seek medical care to rule out something more serious going on. But if it gets worse as the day progresses, settles during the night or is aggravated by meals, your bloating is most likely related to IBS.

Pain

Pain in the abdominal region is a fundamental feature of IBS and is, on average, present for about three days a week, but it can also be a daily problem.[25,26] Abdominal pain can be due to a number of other causes, but IBS-related pain has some characteristic features. IBS pain is sometimes relieved by a bowel movement and may be related to changes in stool frequency or appearance, such as in diarrhoea or constipation,[27] and a common finding is tenderness in the left lower region of the abdomen upon touch.[28] IBS pain is frequently worse after eating, probably due to the normal muscle contractions that occur when digesting food.[29] Research has discovered that the majority of people with IBS have greatly enhanced sensitivity in the gut so that when the gut is distended by the normal passage of food or gas, they experience pain and discomfort when a person without IBS would not.[30]

The chronic, persistent pain of IBS can have a profound effect on your whole body. When you experience pain a signal is relayed through sensory nerve cells in your gut, up into your spinal cord and to your brain. Over time, frequent pain signalling can create changes in the way you process pain that influence pain perception throughout your body and leaves you in a state of chronic hypersensitivity to things that should not be painful, such as food in your digestive system or physical touch.[31]

The fundamental biological purpose of pain is to warn you of danger, such as when you are injured or if you held your finger over a candle flame. Normally pain, which is a response in your brain, not your finger, warns you of the threat and you would instinctively and quickly move your finger to avoid the pain of getting burned. In IBS, however, it's as if your gut is constantly sending this alarm signal to your brain, so you could liken this hypersensitivity to being stuck in a state of constant alarm.

In a striking experiment it was shown that people with IBS have increased sensitivity to heat in their hands and feet, suggesting widespread pain sensitivity, not just in the gut.[32] This might be why people with IBS often report extensive muscle pain, arthritis, headaches, migraines, back pain and neck pain[33] and why approximately one in three people with fibromyalgia, a disease characterized by widespread chronic muscle pain and fatigue, also have IBS.[34]

Although widespread pain is often a part of IBS, in some cases it may be that musculoskeletal problems are causing your pain. A trapped nerve in your spine, for example, can trigger digestive pain. If coughing, sneezing or taking a deep breath, bending, sitting, lifting, twisting or turning over in bed makes your pain worse, there is a good chance it is musculoskeletal. Also, musculoskeletal pain does not tend to be aggravated by eating, or be related to changes in bowel movements typical of IBS. If you think you might have musculoskeletal pain consider seeing a physiotherapist or osteopath.[35]

Pain also takes a powerful psychological toll and is associated with depression, an inability to work and poor quality of life. Some common consequences of chronic pain include:

- fatigue
- disturbed sleep
- poor appetite
- dependence on medication
- overdependence on family
- poor performance on the job or inability to work
- isolation from society and family
- anxiety, fear, bitterness and frustration.[36]

As well as pain causing stress, stress can cause pain. The same regions in your brain that process feelings of pain are also responsible for emotions, such as anger, sadness, fear and anxiety.[37] Because of this crossover between emotions and pain processing, you may find that your pain also varies depending on how you feel.

Beyond your gut

There are a number of general complaints commonly associated with IBS that extend beyond classic gastrointestinal symptoms. These include constant tiredness, backache, headache, an unpleasant taste in the mouth, nausea, vomiting, difficulty swallowing and urinary problems such as needing to go frequently including at night, incomplete emptying of the bladder and painful urination.[38]

One of the interesting things about IBS is that there is usually an overlap of symptoms with other illnesses, which has led some scientists to suggest that this connection is not by chance and what were once thought to be different diseases could actually be symptoms of the same underlying problems. For example, the hypersensitivity in the gut of people with IBS, which is in part responsible for abdominal pain, may not be localized to the gut at all and could be affecting other parts of the body such as your muscles (e.g. back pain) or urinary system (e.g. painful urination). Most certainly some of the underlying features of IBS, such as hypersensitivity in the gut, could also be related to the development of other symptoms or illnesses.

Illnesses that are very common in people with IBS include:

- fibromyalgia: present in 30 to 70 per cent of people with symptoms including muscle tenderness, pain and fatigue[39-41]
- chronic fatigue syndrome: present in 35 to 92 per cent of people with symptoms including chronic, debilitating fatigue

- gastro-oesophageal reflux disease (GORD): present in 19 to 25 per cent of people with symptoms including reflux, heartburn and upper gastrointestinal pain
- chronic pelvic pain syndrome: present in 14 to 79 per cent of people with symptoms including long-term, unexplained disabling pain in the pelvic region[42]
- temporomandibular joint disorder: present in up to 64 per cent of people with symptoms including jaw pain, difficulty chewing and headaches[43]
- functional dyspepsia (gastritis): present in 29 to 87 per cent of people with symptoms including pain in the upper abdomen, feeling of fullness, belching and heartburn[44]
- depression: present in up to 29 per cent of people with symptoms including sadness, hopelessness and loss of interest in daily activities[45]
- anxiety: present in 16.5 to 47 per cent of people with symptoms including worry, fear, irritability and insomnia.[46,47]

Mood and behavioural problems such as depression and anxiety are very common in IBS. Stressful life events can give rise to the development of IBS and stress often makes symptoms worse. The burden of IBS itself can, of course, be very stressful but there is a twist to the relationship between your mood and IBS.

As mentioned earlier, the human gut and brain are connected by your nervous system and can influence each other's function. The old term 'gut feelings' has more merit than is often appreciated. The gastrointestinal changes that underlie IBS may directly influence your mood and behaviour.[48] Quite remarkably, it has been shown that some of the changes in gut function associated with IBS are able to activate the areas of your brain that influence your mood and generate feelings of anxiety.[49] That is not to say that all stress and anxiety could be blamed on your gut, but certainly the line that separates the diagnosis of depression, anxiety and IBS is very blurred. They may be part of the same picture, and your emotions could be affected by your gut health.

Sexual problems are also very common in people with IBS, with up to 40 per cent reporting concerns such as low libido, pain on sexual activity, and worsening of their IBS symptoms following sex.[50] One of the major reasons IBS affects sexual health is that bowel problems directly interfere with sexual activity and can cause people to avoid sex altogether.

It is important to understand that these diverse symptoms and illnesses form part of the bigger picture of IBS, because it could save you from an incorrect diagnosis, the wrong treatment and even unnecessary surgery. A lack of understanding of IBS by medical specialists may lead them to think it's something it's not.

Specialists tend to label people with IBS according to what they know, which is an inherent danger when treating IBS. As you can see, the symptoms are diverse and cross a lot of different body systems, so a rheumatologist who specializes in bones and muscles could diagnose you with fibromyalgia instead of IBS, or a psychologist who works with mood and behaviour could label you with an anxiety disorder. Not seeing the forest for the trees could spell poor treatment. For example, pain in the pelvic region, which is common in IBS, may be misdiagnosed as a gynaecological problem and result in unnecessary surgery.

Unnecessary surgery is a very real problem for people with IBS. One study reported that the rate for back surgery was 50 per cent higher, removal of the appendix or ovaries was 200 per cent higher, and gall-bladder removal was 300 per cent higher in people with IBS.[51] Many of these operations are due to the misdiagnosis of symptoms and, in addition to being unnecessary, only add to the stress and burden of living with IBS.[52]

While the Rome III criteria of bloating and pain with diarrhoea and/or constipation is the textbook definition of IBS, the symptoms are much more diverse and often extend beyond the gastrointestinal tract. These basic symptoms have a lot of nuances and variations, and form part of a much bigger constellation of complaints that can affect your whole mind and body.

WARNING SIGNS OF IBS

There are some important exceptions to the basic symptoms of IBS that may require further investigation to rule out the possibility of other illnesses. If you have IBS symptoms in the presence of one or more of the following warning signs you should seek urgent medical care:

- stools with a very dark black colour or visible blood
- anaemia or low blood-iron levels
- recent, unintentional weight loss
- fever
- family history of ovarian or colon cancer
- symptoms after age 50
- a major change in symptoms.[53,54]

It is important to note that just because you have any of these symptoms does not mean there is actually another underlying illness. In a study of some 1500 people with clinically diagnosed IBS, most people (84 per cent) reported having one or more of these symptoms but only 7 to 9 per cent turned out to have an underlying disease such as colon cancer (0.7 per cent) or Inflammatory Bowel Disease (1.2 per cent),[55] but to be on the safe side you need to speak to your doctor.

If your IBS symptoms started after age 50 you should go for a screening test such as a colonoscopy to rule out colon cancer.[56] In fact, if you are over 50 and haven't had a routine screen for colon cancer you should have one regardless of when your symptoms started. Screening is widely recommended and early detection could literally save your life.

3

WHAT'S GOING ON IN YOUR GUT?

For years IBS has been considered an enigma because there are no conventional medical tests that can accurately diagnose it. This has wrongly led to the assumption that there is nothing fundamentally wrong in having IBS, or worse, that it's psychosomatic or all in your head.

The reality is that there are a number of common underlying functional problems in the digestive, immune and nervous systems of IBS sufferers; it's just that they are difficult to detect and vary from person to person.

One of the reasons these functional problems are often overlooked is that they are difficult to identify with conventional medical testing. Some of the abnormalities are subtle and can't be easily assessed without using techniques that are limited to use in experimental research.

Also, some useful testing techniques are not commonly used in conventional medical practice. There are a number of lesser-known tests that can help identify some of the functional problems in IBS but these are not often used, perhaps due to lack of knowledge, cost or limitations in medical practice guidelines.

Another issue is that not all people with IBS share the same functional gut disturbances. This, of course, makes a strict diagnosis using medical testing impossible and has led to the dismissal of routine investigations, which are seen as costly and unhelpful in making a diagnosis. But what this dismissal fails to take into account is that while testing may not be able to fit everyone with IBS into a diagnostic box, certain tests may be very useful for helping individuals understand what is contributing to their unique illness.

In any case, even without testing, it is helpful to know what is going on in your gut. The functional disturbances that underlie IBS help explain the type and nature of your symptoms and will provide insight into understanding the various causes of IBS and how different treatments work later on.

VISCERAL HYPERSENSITIVITY

Your digestive system is able to sense the contractions and distention that occur as you digest food and is able to do this because the wall of your gastrointestinal tract, like the palm of your hand, contains the sensory receptors that enable you to feel.

Sensory information generated in the gut, such as feeling hunger or fullness, is sent directly to your brain through a kind of gut–brain information highway called the vagus nerve. The primary purpose of the vagus nerve is to communicate between your gut and brain, and vice versa, which is important because your brain and nervous system control many digestive functions.[1]

The same sensory receptors we use to feel can also communicate pain signals when we are exposed to potentially dangerous stimuli such as heat or injury, which you would have experienced if you have ever accidentally burnt yourself. However, in most people with IBS, the pain receptors are in a state of constant hypersensitivity, which helps explain why pain is a characteristic feature of IBS. This constant hypersensitivity of the pain receptors is what is refered to as 'visceral hypersensitivity'.

A number of studies have found that distention of the gut or physical examination of the abdominal area in people with IBS triggers a greatly heightened pain response compared to people who are IBS free. This provides evidence that pain receptors are in a constant state of alarm.

If the same hypersensitivity that occurs in the IBS gut affected the pain receptors in your hands, it would be comparable to feeling pain every time you touched something.

This heightened gut sensitivity is thought to be in part responsible for the urgency of bowel movements, bloating and abdominal pain experienced in IBS, and has also been linked to symptoms beyond the gut.

In addition, this hypersensitivity may not be limited to the gut and is thought to explain why many people with IBS experience wide-ranging pain all over the body, including in the joints, back, neck, muscles and urinary system.[2]

Exactly why hypersensitivity develops is uncertain but it is mostly likely caused by inflammation due to triggers such as infection, stress or dietary factors, and once established remains even when the initial triggers are gone.[3]

DELAYED GASTRIC EMPTYING

A number of people with IBS (about 30 per cent) have delayed gastric emptying, which is a functional problem where the stomach contents are emptied slower than normal. When you eat food, nerve signals cause your stomach muscles to contract to move the food down into your intestines for digestion, but in delayed gastric emptying this process is slowed and the build-up of food can cause digestive problems.

Usually, delayed gastric emptying is caused by nerve damage, which can occur as a complication of diabetes or after abdominal surgery, but in IBS it is thought to be due to a disruption of nerve signals to the stomach.

Delayed gastric emptying has been found to be especially common in people who also suffer from constipation, feeling too full or nausea after eating, or who experience symptoms of heartburn, reflux and dyspepsia.[4] And it is thought that the build-up of food in the gastrointestinal tract may explain these symptoms.

Electrical nerve impulses are what normally trigger muscle contraction and healthy gastric emptying when you are digesting food. However, people with delayed gastric emptying have reduced electrical activity of the stomach muscles, which reduces muscle contractions and delays gastric emptying.[5]

Interestingly, emotions may also play a role in delayed gastric emptying. A study investigating the effects of emotions on gut function found that feelings of anger reduced stomach muscle function in people with IBS.[6] However, it is uncertain whether emotions such as anger are the sole cause of delayed gastric emptying, as it is also possible that they are simply exacerbating the underlying problem.

BACTERIAL OVERGROWTH

Your gut is home to an immense population of bacteria, a population so large they outnumber the cells that comprise your body 10 to 1. Gut bacteria play a critical role in determining the health of your digestive system and disturbances in gut bacteria have been strongly linked to IBS.[7]

In a healthy digestive system, the majority of your gut bacteria reside in your colon or large bowel. However, these bacteria can overgrow into the small intestine, in a condition known as small intestinal bacterial overgrowth (SIBO). A sizeable portion of people with IBS also have SIBO, which may be the cause of their symptoms.

The gut bacteria in your colon play an important role in the digestion of food but if they overpopulate into your small intestine, where they shouldn't be, you start digesting fats and carbohydrates far too early in the digestive process and this can cause fermentation and malabsorption, which can lead to bloating, distention, discomfort and abdominal pain, constipation and diarrhoea.[8]

In addition to SIBO, people with IBS seem to have different gut bacteria compared to people who are IBS free.[9] Specifically, there appear to be higher levels of unhealthy types of bacteria that can cause digestive dysfunction, while the healthy bacteria, especially bifidobacteria, that are normally present and protect against digestive illness, are reduced. If your gut bacterial ecosystem were a garden, the weeds are overtaking the flowers. Emerging evidence suggests that these differences could be due to factors known to cause an imbalance in the gut bacteria such as diet, stress, antibiotics and infection.[10]

Bacterial imbalance can profoundly change the way your gut functions. Gut bacteria communicate directly with your immune and nervous systems, which means a bacterial imbalance has the potential to influence important gut functions such as muscle contractions and pain sensitivity.[11]

Changes in your gut bacteria may also lead to an overgrowth of bad bacteria that are associated with gut problems. For this reason many of the symptoms of IBS could be due to bacterial imbalance and for some people this may be the underlying cause of their problem.[12]

INFLAMMATION

If you have ever accidently cut yourself you will know what inflammation is first-hand — pain, redness and swelling, inflammation is your immune system reacting to an injury or threat to your survival.

The rapid, aggressive inflammation you experience in response to injury is acute and typically short-lived. However, a lingering, subtle inflammation you can't see or feel can also occur in your body and this is exactly what is happening in IBS — the gastrointestinal tissues are in a constant state of low-grade inflammation. Though the inflammation in IBS cannot easily be assessed with conventional tests, a number of research studies have shown that the gastrointestinal tract of people with IBS has much higher levels of immune cells than people who are IBS free, which is indicative of a chronic, low-grade inflammatory state.[13]

Normally, the inflammatory response serves the important purpose of defence and repair, but if it is sustained over long periods of time, even at a low level, immune cells can start to damage and affect the function of surrounding tissues and organs. Low-grade inflammation in gastrointestinal tissue can wreak havoc.

Immune cells are not normally present in high concentrations in the nerve and muscle tissue of the gut, but when they are they can change muscular and sensory nerve function. In fact, immune cells are able to exert such a strong influence because one of their major roles in the gut is to protect you from food-borne infection, in which case they enter the gut and work quickly to cause diarrhoea and the expulsion of contaminated food.

Chronic inflammation, however, means you have loads of immune cells in your gut, all the time pulling their strings on the same muscular and nerve cells, and that's when things start to go wrong. The major cause of increased gut-pain sensitivity in IBS is thought to be inflammation. Biopsies of the gut tissue of people with IBS have found that inflammatory immune cells are constantly exciting nerve endings in the gut tissue and that is why the gut is so sensitive and painful.[14]

Immune cells can also directly influence muscle function and therefore inflammation helps explain the increased or decreased gut transit time that accompanies diarrhoea and constipation, as well as alterations in muscle contractions linked to bloating and distention.[15]

Because inflammation may be due to a host of factors such as diet, stress and infection it is not exactly clear why the IBS gut is inflamed and the reason could vary from person to person. However, one of the most likely candidates is gut bacteria. An examination of the gastrointestinal tissue of IBS sufferers has identified an unusual increase in cellular receptors that recognize bad bacteria in your gut and trigger inflammation by activating your immune system.[16]

INTESTINAL PERMEABILITY

From your mouth right to the other end of your gastrointestinal tract there is a connected barrier of cells that separates you from the 'outside world' — your gut wall. Your gut wall is key to keeping your gastric contents where they should be — in your gastrointestinal tract. If the contents of your gut pass into your bloodstream they can evoke inflammation, both locally in your gut wall and even systemically throughout your whole body.[17]

Intestinal permeability, also known as leaky gut, can occur due to direct damage to the gut wall or through increases in the size of the junctions between the cells that line the gut wall.[18] Importantly, the gut wall does not form a tight impermeable seal, otherwise you would not be able to absorb nutrients from food. Rather, the junctions between cells are to some extent naturally 'leaky'. This leakiness, however, can be increased by a number of things including unhealthy diets, alcohol, gut infections, anti-inflammatory medications and stress.[19]

A number of studies have found evidence that some people with IBS have leaky gut. Leaky gut seems to particularly affect people with diarrhoea-predominant and post-infectious IBS and is thought to be due to increased inflammation in the gastrointestinal tissue.

The severity of leaky gut has also been correlated with the level of reported pain in IBS sufferers, suggesting it plays a direct role in symptoms.[20] Leaky gut allows a flood of substances from your gut, including food allergens and bacteria, to enter your gut wall, which can activate inflammation.[21] And this inflammatory response could create a constant stimulation of pain receptors in your gut and all the way up your spinal cord into your brain, leading to chronic pain and sensitivity.

People with IBS and intestinal permeability have been shown

to have higher pain sensitivity beyond the gut as well. One interesting study found that intestinal permeability correlated with a sensitivity test (applied heat) on the calf muscle of the lower leg, suggesting that leaky gut may be linked to the wider pain symptoms often experienced by IBS sufferers.[22]

Interestingly, intestinal permeability seems to be more common in people with IBS who also have allergic diseases such as eczema, asthma or hay fever.[23] It may be that the contents of the gut, which include food particles and inhaled pollen, passing through a leaky gut wall, increases your risk of developing allergic responses to certain foods and airborne allergens.

STRESS

The lining of your gastrointestinal tract is embedded with a nervous system called the enteric nervous system, also known as the 'little brain'. The enteric nervous system was discovered in the nineteenth century and was a breakthrough in understanding the connection between the brain and the gut, or what is now referred to as the gut–brain axis.

The gut–brain axis is actually made up of a wide range of hormones and nerve pathways that collectively create a communication network between your gut and your brain. Your brain and nervous system control many important functions of your gastrointestinal tract, including secretions of stomach acid and digestive enzymes as well as muscle contractions. So as you might imagine, changes in your thoughts and feelings, such as when you are under stress, can also change your gut function.

Stress has long been known to influence digestive function and a vast amount of research in this area has linked stress to many of the major gut disturbances found in IBS including inflammation, increased gut permeability, hypersensitivity to pain and changes in gastric emptying.[24]

Stress can, of course, affect gut function in everyone but people with IBS are much more sensitive to the effects of stress and have been shown in a number of studies to have greater changes in gut motility, pain perception and emotional symptoms and have an amplified production of stress hormones compared to people who are IBS free.[25]

While stress can trigger and exacerbate the symptoms of IBS, it is also true that gut dysfunction can actually be a source of stress itself. Inflammation, bad gut bacteria, increased pain perception and intestinal permeability can all chronically activate your nervous system and increase the physical and emotional symptoms of stress.[26] For example, a remarkable experimental study demonstrated that gut bacteria are able to directly communicate with your brain via the vagus nerve, which runs between your brain and gastrointestinal tract. In this study, the administration of a probiotic supplement of beneficial gut bacteria was able to relieve anxiety through stimulation of the vagus nerve.[27]

It is important to understand that the brain–gut connection in IBS is a two-way street, with stress influencing gut dysfunction, and gut dysfunction being a source of stress. This does not mean that IBS is a stress-related or psychological disorder; rather, it means that the brain and gut are intimately interconnected and gut symptoms, such as abdominal pain, can go hand-in-hand with brain symptoms, such as anxiety.

PART 2

HOW TO ACHIEVE GREAT GUT HEALTH

4

BANISH BAD BUGS AND BALANCE YOUR BACTERIA

The 1 to 1.5 kilograms (2–3 lb) of bacteria that reside in the human gut are so vast that they outnumber the cells in the human body 10 to 1. In fact, this immense bacterial mass has been likened to a vital organ, which is similar in size to your liver and just as important.

Your gut bacteria form a huge microbial ecosystem that performs many vital roles such as maintenance of a healthy immune system, digestion of food, production of vitamins, detoxification of toxic compounds and prevention of the overgrowth of harmful gut bacteria. Most importantly, your gut bacteria keep your digestive system functioning well through their influence on digestive processes.

The disruption of healthy gut flora has been termed 'dysbiosis', which refers to an imbalance or overgrowth of bad bacteria in your gut that results in dysfunction or disease. Several factors associated with our modern lifestyles have been linked to the development of dysbiosis, including the use of antibiotics, psychological stress and unhealthy diets.[1]

There is strong evidence to suggest that dysbiosis is a major cause of digestive problems. In particular, there are two major disturbances of the gut bacteria that have been blamed: an increase in the number of bacteria in the small bowel, known as small intestinal bacterial overgrowth (SIBO); and an increased level of bad bacteria and decreased level of good bacteria in the colon or large bowel.[2] Infections with bacteria or parasites from contaminated food or water can also play an important role, but this is more often an initial trigger rather than an ongoing underlying problem.

SMALL INTESTINAL BACTERIAL OVERGROWTH

In a healthy digestive system the majority of your gut bacteria reside in your colon or large bowel. However, these bacteria can overgrow into the small intestine and cause small intestinal bacterial overgrowth (SIBO).

A sizeable portion of people with IBS also have SIBO, which may in fact be the cause of their symptoms. One study found that, when tested, 84 per cent of its subjects with IBS had higher fermentation and gas production, which is an indicator of SIBO. In the same study, the subjects were treated with an antibiotic that is not absorbed into the bloodstream but remains in the gut and kills off the bacterial overgrowth. Remarkably this resulted in a 75 per cent improvement in all of their symptoms.[3] In two larger follow-up studies, treatment for two weeks with a non-absorbable antibiotic resulted in significant improvement in IBS symptoms and bloating compared to placebo and the effects were still present at a follow-up visit ten weeks later.[4] These studies are compelling evidence that for some people SIBO is a real and treatable cause of IBS.

Normally, bacteria in the colon ferment dietary carbohydrates such as sugars and fibre. This fermentation is part of the digestive process and feeds the good bacteria in your gut that are vital for your health. Fermentation, as the term might suggest, can result in the production of gas, which is not normally a problem (apart from social embarrassment perhaps) but when SIBO is present carbohydrates are fermented much earlier than usual in the abdominal region, which can then result in excessive gas building up in the small intestine resulting in bloating, distention, discomfort and abdominal pain.[5]

The bacteria present in SIBO are not only good at digesting carbohydrates to make gas, they are great at breaking down fats as well. Fats are normally eliminated from your body by your gall bladder, which produces bile salts that bind fats, allowing their easy elimination through your digestive system. The bile-busting bacteria that are overgrowing in the digestive system of people with SIBO, however, can break down these bile salts, releasing the fats from their salts, causing fatty diarrhoea and discomfort.[6]

People with SIBO also tend to have higher overall levels of bad bacteria including *Escherichia coli* (*E. coli*), *Enterococcus* and *Klebsiella pneumoniae*.[7] Overgrowth of these bad bugs results in the production of bacterial toxins, which can activate your immune system causing damage to your gut wall, inflammation, increased sensitivity, pain, constipation and diarrhoea.[8] A study in elderly people with SIBO found that their gut walls were damaged and thinned; this destruction was most certainly a direct result of bacterial overgrowth because after they were treated with antibiotics and the overgrowth was eliminated their gut walls healed and returned to normal.[9]

Symptoms of SIBO

The symptoms of SIBO are mainly related to the excessive production of gas in the small intestine. SIBO may also cause symptoms that are not often thought of as being related to digestive health, including skin problems (rosacea) and muscular pain and chronic fatigue (fibromyalgia).

The most common symptoms of SIBO include:

- bloating
- flatulence
- abdominal discomfort
- diarrhoea
- abdominal pain.

The less common symptoms of SIBO are:

- weight loss
- fatty, oily or floating faeces (steatorrhoea)
- facial redness and acne (rosacea)
- arthritic pains
- anaemia
- nerve pain due to vitamin B12 deficiency
- fatigue and muscle pain (fibromyalgia)
- coeliac disease
- lactose intolerance.[10-17]

What causes SIBO?

A well-functioning digestive system normally prevents the overgrowth of bacteria in the small intestine through natural defences such as stomach acid and the muscular contractions that move food through your digestive system, but when these are under-functioning or disrupted, SIBO can develop.

One of the major functions of stomach acid, apart from helping you digest food, is to act as an antibacterial buffer to prevent gut infections, so low stomach-acid production is a major reason for bacterial overgrowth. Your stomach acid could be low for a number of reasons, the most common being due to the use of antacids, increasing age and a condition known as atrophic gastritis, a disorder of chronic inflammation in the upper gastrointestinal tract.

Even short use of the antacid medication called proton-pump inhibitors (PPIs) has been shown to lower gastric acid, cause bacterial overgrowth and affect digestive health.[18] While antacids are not always to blame, the fact that antacids can cause SIBO and are commonly used by people with IBS suggests that antacid use may have a lot to do with IBS for some people.[19]

A study in which subjects experiencing reflux were given a proton-pump inhibitor and their symptoms monitored for more than six months, found that after eight weeks of treatment 43 per cent complained of bloating and other common side effects including flatulence, abdominal pain and diarrhoea. Six months later 26 per cent had developed SIBO and a significant number had also developed IBS.[20]

Atrophic gastritis can also dramatically reduce stomach acid production. The chance that you might have atrophic gastritis gets higher as you age, with some 50 per cent of people over the age of 60 estimated to suffer from the disease.[21] One of the most common causes of atrophic gastritis is infection with the bacteria *Helicobacter pylori*, which can be treated with antibiotics.

In addition to stomach acid, the normal passage of food through your gut keeps bacterial overgrowth at bay. As you digest food, smooth muscles along the digestive tract move the food matter along in an action called gut motility. Reductions in gut motility may cause a build-up of food in the small intestine, allowing it to ferment and cause bacterial overgrowth. Older age is associated with low gut motility and older people are more likely to have SIBO. Constipation, a common symptom of IBS, is also associated with low gut motility and may be a cause of SIBO too.[22]

Gluten intolerance has also been linked to SIBO, most likely because when you eat gluten it triggers an immune response that damages the gut wall and its defences, leading to bacterial overgrowth. Interestingly, people with coeliac disease on a gluten-free diet may continue to have the digestive symptoms of gluten sensitivity despite eliminating the cause (gluten) because SIBO is still causing problems.[23] However, if you have coeliac disease and go on a gluten-free diet your gut wall will start to heal and eventually return to normal, which may be enough to eliminate SIBO with time.[24]

INCREASED LEVELS OF BAD BACTERIA AND IBS

For some years disturbances in gut bacteria have been thought to play a role in the development of IBS but only recently has the scientific research really strengthened our understanding of this relationship. Various lines of evidence have shown that changes in gut bacteria, such as an overgrowth of bad bacteria and a decline in good bacteria, could result in an inflammatory response in the gut that can cause many of the symptoms of IBS.[25]

One of the most common findings in the gut of people with IBS is a decline in bifidobacteria, with several recent studies suggesting this is very often the case.[26] Bifidobacteria are normally a predominant species of bacteria in the gastrointestinal tract and are responsible for many of the health effects of the gut flora, including the production of vitamins, detoxification of toxic substances, maintenance of a healthy immune response, and the prevention of the overgrowth of bad bacteria. So it makes sense then that if your bifidobacteria are low you are going to be in trouble.

There is direct evidence to suggest that declines in bifidobacteria could result in IBS symptoms. A revealing study from Finland set out to see if changes in gut flora were linked to digestive problems, by monitoring gut bacterial populations in the gastrointestinal tract and reporting symptoms over a seven-week period. Over this time some of the subjects had important changes in their gut bacteria that correlated with the use of antibiotics, overseas travel and temporary illness — factors all known to have a strong effect on the balance of gut bacteria. The most striking finding from this study was that those subjects who reported abdominal pain had a five-fold decrease in bifidobacteria levels compared to those subjects who had no pain or change in their gut flora.[27]

A number of studies have also found that in addition to lower levels of bifidobacteria, people with IBS have many other differences in their gut flora compared to people who are IBS free.[28] For instance, there may be higher levels of nasty pathogenic bacteria such as *Clostridium difficile* and *Staphylococcus aureus*.[29,30] But the distinction between the bacterial ecosystem of a healthy gut and the gut of someone with IBS is complex and far from clear. There are over 1000 bacterial species in the human gut, making it the most diverse bacterial ecosystem on Earth. Because of this incredible diversity, simple clear-cut differences in the gut bacteria of IBS sufferers are unlikely.[31]

Further evidence that gut bacteria play a fundamental role in IBS comes from studies of probiotics. Probiotics are beneficial bacteria that are used as a dietary supplement, and have been extensively studied in people with IBS. The concept behind probiotic therapy is that by consuming good bacteria you can influence the overall health of your gut ecology, increasing the overall levels of desirable bacteria and reducing the bad ones, a bit like weeding and feeding a garden.

Some probiotic bacteria have produced remarkable results in IBS sufferers. One such study of the probiotic *Lactobacillus plantarum* 299v found that it was able to significantly reduce pain and improve constipation and bloating within just four weeks, with 95 per cent of people reporting benefits.[32] Studies such as this not only provide strong evidence for the very important role of bacterial imbalance in IBS, but also offer hope for a new and effective avenue of treatment with probiotics.

Post-infectious IBS

One of the most common triggers of IBS is an acute gastrointestinal infection, such as traveller's diarrhoea or food poisoning. In fact, about one in three people with IBS can trace the onset back to such an illness. If you had a bout of infectious illness like this you probably know about it; acute infection causes diarrhoea, abdominal cramps, increased stool frequency, bloody or mucousy stools and weight loss.

The more severe the symptoms and the longer their duration, the higher your chances are of developing post-infectious IBS. For example, if you have diarrhoea for one week, your risk increases by 200 per cent and if the diarrhoea continues for three weeks so does your risk, shooting up to 300 per cent. But it is not just diarrhoea that increases your risk; the presence of weight loss and bloody stools and especially abdominal cramps also raise your chances of developing IBS.[33]

Post-infectious IBS is not just a continuation of your symptoms either; in fact your illness might completely resolve, only for IBS to develop many months or even years later. Even if you had a bout of illness and recovered, you are still at a high risk of developing IBS for up to three years after the initial infection.[34]

A range of infectious bacteria have been implicated in post-infectious IBS including *Campylobacter*, *Clostridium perfringens*, *Clostridium difficile*, *Staphylococcus aureus*, *salmonella* and *Escherichia coli*.[35] Parasitic infection with *Giardia lamblia* (giardiasis) has also been strongly linked to the subsequent development of IBS.[36] These nasty organisms are generally contracted through exposure to contaminated food and water, especially in developing countries where hygiene standards may be lower, although food poisoning is certainly not uncommon in developed countries as well.

A well-studied outbreak of *Giardia lamblia* in the city of Bergen, Norway, is an excellent example of just how devastating the infection can be. In 2004 there was a large-scale outbreak of giardia due to unusually heavy rainfall, which caused sewage to overflow into a lake that supplied drinking water to the city centre. The result was an estimated 2500 people developing giardiasis.[37] Thankfully the outbreak was detected and brought under control with antibiotic treatment, but unlike giardia outbreaks in other countries, scientists in Norway have been closely studying many of the people who were affected to see what the long-term effects on digestive health are, and the results are rather alarming.

Almost half the people who were infected during the outbreak are thought to have developed post-infectious IBS. To see how bad the symptoms were, a group of just over 80 people who developed ongoing digestive problems were called in to have their symptoms assessed two to three years after they had been treated for giardia. Most of them had textbook IBS with severe bloating, diarrhoea and abdominal pain. They also commonly reported that their symptoms were worse after eating certain foods or when stressed. Also, a particularly striking discovery was the number of people from the initial outbreak who now had chronic debilitating fatigue — some 46 per cent of people three years after the initial outbreak.[38,39]

It is thought that acute gastrointestinal infections, whether they are due to a parasite such as *Giardia lamblia* or a bacteria such as *E. coli*, set you up for IBS because of the havoc they wreak on your gastrointestinal tract. Acute inflammation, changes in your gut bacteria, alterations in gut motility and increases in intestinal permeability take hold during the infection and don't resolve easily once the infection has gone.[40] This leaves you open and vulnerable to developing IBS.

PARASITE INFECTION

A commonly overlooked cause of chronic digestive issues is infection with a parasite, and the reason it is often overlooked is because the scientific evidence linking contribution of parasites recent and both relatively new is not widely known.

Infection with a parasite can be very serious, causing symptoms such as chronic and severe diarrhoea with rapid weight loss. But there are subtler types of infection, the symptoms of which are less severe and could mimic those of IBS. Such symptoms are less obviously due to a parasite and one of the reasons why infection may be overlooked as a cause of your digestive issues. Another reason is that, historically, the main parasite associated with IBS was generally considered not to play a role, but recent research has turned that dismissal on its head.

A peculiar family of parasites long associated with chronic digestive issues are the *Blastocystis* species. *Blastocystis* is peculiar because many people carry this parasite but have no symptoms, and because of this fact early studies sometimes found no link between *Blastocystis* and gastrointestinal problems, subsequently dismissing it as unimportant.[41] However, in recent years a large amount of research with more sophisticated technology has demonstrated that infection with *Blastocystis* is linked to symptoms in some people and we also now understand why some suffer while other people do not.[42]

One of the more rigorous and recent studies on *Blastocystis* helps shed some light on the link to IBS. A French research team set out to compare differences in *Blastocystis* infection between people with IBS and those who were symptom free; they also looked at whether or not *Blastocystis* was linked to imbalance in gut bacteria. In addition, they conducted an analysis of all the existing studies to date and published these findings in the major journal, *Public Library of Science*.[43] In their study they found that the highest prevalence of *Blastocystis* was in the people with IBS, but this was not much more than people who were symptom-free (23.2 per cent versus 16.1 per cent). This is a curious finding but we will explore why this might be in a moment. They also revealed that there were some important differences in gut bacteria associated with *Blastocystis*, including a reduction in bacteria associated with better digestive health, such as bifidobacteria. And finally, when they reviewed eleven existing studies looking at associations between *Blastocystis* and IBS they demonstrated that, collectively, infection is 2.34 times more common in patients with IBS than not. All of this points to infection as a cause of IBS, by why would some people have symptoms and not others?

There are a few plausible reasons why *Blastocystis* could cause symptoms for some people but not others, with one of the most likely being that there are a number of different subtypes of the parasite and that some are problematic while others are not and could simply be a normal part of your gut ecosystem. There have been thirteen subtypes of *Blastocystis* documented, with some subtypes more strongly associated with gastrointestinal symptoms.[44] One reason for this is that different subtypes of *Blastocystis* may have different characteristics that render them problematic, such as better ability to cause inflammation, intestinal permeability or disruption to your gut bacteria.[45]

These new discoveries still leave us with the questions: is *Blastocystis* a cause of my symptoms? And if it is, what can I do about it? Unfortunately, there is no clear answer to these questions yet. Because it is hard to be certain if *Blastocystis* is causing your symptoms or is just an innocent bystander, the decision to treat it is often down to the best decision of your gastroenterologist and typically decided after ruling out all other possible causes. Further complicating matters, *Blastocystis* is known to disappear of its own accord. In one study of 100 people with *Blastocystis*, all patients improved and in 91.2 per cent of them the parasite was no longer detectable after one year, without any treatment.[46]

CANDIDA OVERGROWTH

Dietary, nutritional and antifungal treatments for chronic candida infection have been used for over 40 years and over this time have been extremely controversial. New research into the role of candida overgrowth, however, may warrant a serious reconsideration of 'the yeast connection'.

Candida is a type of yeast and many harmless species normally live in your digestive system; however, some species can be harmful and they can also overgrow or in extreme cases invade your body and cause serious illness. Critical illness due to candida is not controversial and is a well-established medical issue. What is controversial is that for many years integrative medicine practitioners have linked a subtler chronic candida infection to symptoms of IBS, other digestive symptoms, allergies and even mental health issues.

Chronic candida infection — also known as candidiasis, or candida hypersensitivity syndrome — was first reported in 1978 when Dr C. Orian Truss described over a decade's experience in treating a wide range of otherwise unexplained symptoms with antifungal medication.[47] This work was then expanded by Dr William Crook who communicated with Truss after noticing improvement in a mutual patient, and then later popularized the treatment of chronic candida infection with a low-sugar diet and antifungal therapy in 1983 with the publication of his book, *The Yeast Connection.*[48]

Chronic candida infection has since attracted considerable criticism by conventional academic medicine,[49,50] yet many clinicians employing anticandida dietary approaches and treatments, including nutritional and herbal medicine, have continued to report important clinical results.[51-54] A problem with chronic candida infection is that much of the research supporting it is now relatively old and often overlooked or discredited as a consequence. However, new research may change that and call for a renaissance of anticandida therapy.

One of the most compelling links between candida overgrowth and digestive problems is related to gastrointestinal inflammation. Although candida species are considered a normal type of fungus in the human gut, healthy individuals tend to harbour very low levels of candida in their colon.[55] But in people with inflammatory bowel disease, there may be an overgrowth of candida that is related to inflammation in their digestive system.

Because candida levels in stool samples (which is what is typically used to measure gut bacteria) are different from those living along the gut wall, investigating the presence of candida is difficult. But a recent study comparing surgically obtained specimens from people with inflammatory bowel disease to healthy people produced some remarkable insights.[56] Laser scanning of the specimens clearly showed a rich and diverse elevation of fungal and candida species in the inflamed gut wall. Further, the mucosal fungal community was associated with higher levels of inflammatory markers both in their gut and in their blood, and more candida was also linked to more clinical symptoms. This is not an isolated study, with other recent reports finding similar links to candida and good clinical responses to anti-fungal treatments.[57]

Although likely to remain controversial for some time, there is important reason to believe that some people might have an overgrowth of candida and that this could be causing gastrointestinal symptoms as well as other problems. In any case, if you have suspected candida overgrowth the same treatments (reducing intake of sugars and taking antimicrobial herbs and probiotics) can be an effective way to improve your gut bacteria and reduce symptoms, as we will see when we look at how to improve your gut bacteria, and in Chapter 8, 'Put your bacteria on a low-carbohydrate diet'.

Are 'bad bugs' the cause of your IBS?

There are a few things you can do to find out if bad bugs are causing your IBS.

1. **Do you have a history of infection?** Think back to when your symptoms started. Did you travel overseas? Even if your symptoms occurred months after getting back home they could still be related to an infection you caught while travelling. You might have also had a short bout of food poisoning or a tummy bug. If you did, chances are your gut bacteria are out of balance and you might even have a parasite such as giardia, so you need to get tested (especially if you have persistent diarrhoea).

2. **Have you used antibiotics?** Antibiotics can have a very disruptive effect on your gut bacteria, killing off the good bugs and letting the bad ones take over. In one study, 33 per cent of people with IBS reported using an antibiotic in the previous year, making it a powerful risk factor for the development of digestive symptoms.[58] If you have taken antibiotics frequently in the past, particularly in the last year, this may help explain why you have IBS.

3. **Test your gut bacteria:** There are tests available that enable you to get a very detailed and clear

picture of the levels of good and bad bacteria in your digestive system. Your doctor might offer you what is called a parasitology test, which looks only for parasites, but this won't give you a comprehensive assessment as it only tests for a few major offenders. The more detailed test is called a comprehensive parasitology profile, which looks at a wide range of parasites and bacteria and is available through specialist functional diagnostic laboratories (see Resources). These are more expensive but will give you a clearer picture of the overall levels of good and bad bacteria in your gastrointestinal tract (such as bifidobacteria and *E. coli*), as well as any possible parasites. The test involves providing three samples of your stools over three consecutive days, which may sound like a tall order, but you are provided with the instructions and equipment you need, making it relatively easy.

4. **Test for small intestinal bacterial overgrowth (SIBO)**: A hydrogen breath test is used to diagnose SIBO. This typically involves eating a low-fibre diet for one day, a twelve-hour overnight fast, then drinking a solution of lactulose or glucose (it doesn't matter too much which one) and having the amount of hydrogen in your breath measured every fifteen minutes over three hours, by breathing into a tube. This test is, however, controversial because of its potential inaccuracy, but it has been used successfully to identify SIBO, help direct treatments that reduce bacterial overgrowth and subsequently reduce symptoms. And a return of a positive breath

test correlates with a return of symptoms. So, regardless of controversy, this is currently the best and most practical way to see if you have SIBO and it is generally reliable.

TAKE THE CANDIDA QUIZ

The identification of candida is mostly based on clinical history and symptoms, as diagnostic tests can lack accuracy.[59] Typical symptoms, along with a history of vaginal yeast infections, oral thrush or previous antibiotic prescriptions, may indicate need for treatment. And a 7-item 'Fungus-related Disease Questionnaire' (FRDQ-7) is sometimes used to identify if you might benefit from treatments and dietary changes.[60]

Fungus-related Disease Questionnaire-7 (FRDQ-7)

Score: 0 = none, 1 = occasional or mild, 2 = frequent or moderately severe, 3 = severe or disabling

- Have you, at any time in your life, taken broad-spectrum antibiotics?
- Have you taken tetracycline or other broad-spectrum antibiotics for one month or longer?
- Are your symptoms worse on damp, muggy days or in mouldy places?
- Do you crave sugar?
- Do you have a feeling of being 'drained' of energy?
- **WOMEN** Are you bothered with vaginal burning, itching or discharge?
- **MEN** Do you have burning, itching or discharge from the penis?
- Are you bothered by burning, itching or tearing of your eyes?

Result: Score 0–3 = a fungus-related disease (FRD) is unlikely; 4–9 = FRD probable; 10–21 = FRD almost certain.

5. **Treat yourself and see what happens:** This may not sound like very professional advice but trying the treatments below might be a simple and effective way to see if bad bugs are the problem. For example, if you respond exceptionally well to a probiotic, chances are that bacterial imbalance was at least in part to blame for your symptoms The methods and tests above, however, are going to give you a much better idea of what's going on and may pick up something serious, like a parasite, that needs to be treated with medication.

HOW TO IMPROVE YOUR GUT BACTERIA

Probiotics

Probiotics are widely claimed to help IBS and while some do, others may not work at all and some can even make things worse. Not all probiotics are the same and it pays to know the difference. For example, one study found that a probiotic supplement actually made symptoms worse, while other studies have shown some probiotics have no effect and others provide relief from only certain symptoms such as bloating.[61-63]

However there are probiotics that can provide substantial overall relief.[64] This is because different probiotic strains may have very different clinical effects. Probiotics are named according to their genus, species and then specific strain:

Lactobacillus (genus), *plantarum* (species), 299v (strain). So, if you are considering using a probiotic for IBS, it pays to use one that has been shown to improve symptoms in a clinical study. The Five Steps to Great Gut Health program has a guide to probiotics that are particularly effective (see page 160).[65]

You may need to do a bit of research to get beyond potentially misleading marketing claims and find a probiotic supplement that has been shown to actually work, but it could be worth the extra effort. When trialling a probiotic give it about four weeks, and if it does not work try a different product to see if a different strain or combination of strains works better for you.

Some probiotics have also been shown to reduce SIBO, though again not all of them seem to be effective.[66] Strains that have shown very promising results include *Lactobacillus casei* Shirota strain (in Yakult), *Bacillus clausii* and *Lactobacillus johnsonii* La1 (in yoghurt and supplements) and a mixture of the following four strains in supplement form: *Lactobacillus casei, Lactobacillus plantarum, Enterococcus faecalis* and *Bifidobacterium brevis*.[67-70] These are typically taken for a course of four to six weeks and have been shown to be as or more effective at eradicating SIBO than antibiotic drugs.

Keep in mind that the effects of probiotics are varied, and sometimes people experience transient bloating or gas over the first two to three days. In addition, most studies have shown that the beneficial effects of probiotic supplements on your gut bacteria don't last after you stop taking them, so you may find you need to take them long term.

Prebiotics

Prebiotics are special types of fibre that feed bifidobacteria and boost their numbers in the gut. Natural sources of prebiotics include acacia gum, inulin (found in Jerusalem artichokes and chicory root), wholegrain oats and unrefined wheat. When you consume prebiotics that can increase the level of good bifidobacteria in your gastrointestinal tract, they competitively kill off the bad bacteria and balance out your gut ecosystem. Prebiotics are therefore associated with wide-ranging health benefits and have been studied in people with IBS.

Research has shown that prebiotics can have negative or positive effects on IBS, depending on the dose. High doses (about 20 g daily) can make symptoms worse, probably because they are fermented and consequently make too much gas, although symptoms do improve after the first few months. Small doses (about 3–5 g daily), however, don't make symptoms worse and have shown the greatest likelihood of benefit, improving flatulence, bloating and overall wellbeing while measurably increasing the proportion of bifidobacteria in the gut.[71] Studies have found significant improvements after six weeks of daily use at this lower dose.

There are many different types of prebiotics available but the ones shown to be beneficial are short-chain fructo-oligosaccharides (found in chicory, asparagus, onion, garlic, banana, artichoke) and galacto-oligosaccharides (found in milk). If you are going to trial prebiotics these are the ones to go for. They are best consumed as dietary supplements so you get the correct daily dose.

Like probiotics, you may get some transient gas or bloating over the first few days and you may also find that you get the best results taking prebiotics long term. It may also help to know that with probiotics and prebiotics, it doesn't matter if you miss a day or two between doses, because their effects are maintained and you will continue to benefit.

Fermented foods

For much of human history we have used fermentation as a way of preserving and improving the nutritional quality of foods. Slow sourdough fermentation helps improve the digestibility, nutritional value and flavour of bread, for example.[72] It also helps reduce digestive problems people might get from eating modern processed bread.[73] But of special interest are the bacteria that these foods contain and the potential of fermented foods to act as natural probiotics and prebiotics.

There are literally hundreds of traditional fermented foods that were used across many different cultures, but sadly these food traditions are being lost to the industrialization of our diets.[74] However there is a fermented food revival occurring as we re-discover the importance of these foods for our health. Fermented foods are not only a source of probiotic bacteria and prebiotic fibres, but also often rich in polyphenols and other bioactive substances produced during fermentation, making them an important part of a healthy diet.[75]

Two fermented foods that have attracted scientific attention in particular are kimchi (Korean fermented vegetables) and kefir (fermented dairy). Importantly, both are teeming with bacteria and have been shown to influence our gut bacteria when we eat them, which is not true for all fermented foods, and makes them good candidates for probiotic health benefits.[76,77] And they have shown some important health effects: for example, in one study, consuming kefir regularly was found to help improve blood sugar metabolism and cholesterol.[78] Eating kimchi regularly had similar beneficial effects, in addition to helping reduce body weight in people who were overweight.[79] It is likely that these benefits are partly the result of improvements in gut bacteria, and there might be benefits to eating them regularly if you have digestive symptoms too.

A number of clinical studies suggest that kefir may have important digestive health benefits, with one study showing it helped to improve lactose digestion in people with lactose intolerance and another in which it was shown to help reduce symptoms in people with bacterial infection also taking antibiotics.[80,81] Kefir can also help improve regularity and reduce digestive discomfort. In one study, people with a history of constipation drank 500 ml (1 pt) a day of kefir for four weeks. At the end of the study there was an improvement in gut transit time, increased stool frequency, improved stool consistency, and decreased laxative use, with 50 per cent of people stopping laxatives completely. The degree of straining during evacuation showed a tendency to improve with kefir, and bowel satisfaction scores also significantly improved.[82]

So consuming traditional fermented foods such as kefir and kimchi, or other such foods that are perhaps more culturally specific to you, could help keep your digestive system healthy by improving your gut bacteria.

Peppermint oil

A number of studies have found that enteric-coated essential peppermint oil capsules can improve the symptoms of IBS, such as diarrhoea, constipation, bloating and pain. In fact, peppermint oil is one of the best-studied natural medicines for IBS.[83]

Peppermint oil seems to work because it reduces muscle spasms and acts as a muscle relaxant; however, it has also been shown to influence your gut bacteria, in particular killing off bad bugs including bacteria, yeasts, fungi and parasites.

Perhaps not surprisingly, there is also some evidence to show that peppermint oil can improve SIBO. A twenty-day course of peppermint oil at a dose of 0.2 ml three times daily has been found to be effective.[84]

It is important to use an enteric-coated product, as the enteric coating stops the breakdown of the capsule in your stomach and delivers the active ingredients to the intestine. If there is no enteric coating the peppermint oil tends to get digested before it has a chance to work, and you are also more likely to get unpleasant, peppermint-flavoured indigestion.

Clinical research suggests that one to two enteric-coated capsules containing 0.2–0.4 ml of peppermint oil taken three times a day for about four weeks can improve IBS symptoms. Mixtures of peppermint with other essential oils may work well too. Unless you have a known allergy to peppermint there are few side effects and it is very safe. Avoid peppermint oil if you are pregnant, and if you are on medication speak to your doctor first.

Herbs for bacterial overgrowth

Although antibiotics are used to treat SIBO, a number of integrative practitioners and medical centres have been using herbal alternatives with similar success. The first documentation of this was published in the journal *Global Advances in Health and Medicine* and suggested that herbal treatment may be safer and more effective than antibiotics for SIBO. This is an important finding for people with chronic digestive symptoms.

In the study, people who had SIBO confirmed with a breath test were treated with either herbal therapy (one of a number of different products) or antibiotics (rifaximin) then had their treatment results reviewed. The rate of successful treatment of SIBO, as confirmed with a follow-up breath test, was 46 per cent in the herbal therapy group compared to 34 per cent in those who received rifaximin. And people who did not respond to rifaximin were offered either a stronger course of three antibiotics or herbal therapy, which were equally effective at eradicating SIBO (both about a 60 per cent successful treatment).[85]

Adverse effects in those taking rifaximin were more common and severe than those receiving herbal therapy, suggesting herbs are a safer option. 'In summary, we conclude that in the setting of SIBO, patients can be given the choice of antibiotic or herbal therapy depending on their individual preference, with similar response rates and safety profiles,' wrote the study investigators. 'In addition, patients who are refractory [do not respond] to rifaximin can receive herbal therapy as a potential rescue therapy with equivalent results to triple antibiotics.'

The people in this study were given one of a number of herbal products containing multiple herbs, and were also given a different product if the first did not work. The dose was two capsules or tablets morning and night, regardless of the product, for four weeks. Each contained several antimicrobial herbs and extracts such as Olive leaf (*Olea europaea*, leaf), Pau D'Arco (inner bark), Oregano (*Origanum vulgare*, essential oil), Thyme (*Thymus vulgaris*, essential oil), Wormwood (*Artemisia absinthium*, shoots and leaves extract) and Berberine. The benefit of using multiple herbs, and multiple products, is that it has more chance of having the desired broad-spectrum antimicrobial effect.

If you have confirmed or suspected SIBO, you could try a four-week course of a good antimicrobial herbal product at a dose of two tablets or capsules twice daily. This is best done under the supervision of a healthcare practitioner but has very low risk of side effects, so you could simply try it and see if it helps. Once you have finished your four-week course it would be advisable to start a good probiotic supplement and continue taking it daily for a few months as your system readjusts. Or if you did not respond to the first course, you could try another four weeks with a different product.

Natural anti-parasitic therapy

The conventional treatment for parasites such as *Blastocystis* typically involves anti-parasitic drugs such as metronidazole, but this does not always work, and the success in eradicating the parasite is anywhere between 0 per cent and 100 per cent in various studies.[86] For this reason many other anti-parasitic drugs may be used, and one approach that has been reported to be particularly effective by the Centre for Digestive Diseases, Sydney, involves three drugs, but this treatment or the medications are not commonly available outside of this treatment centre.[87]

One potential problem with metronidazole is that it may increase chances of *Blastocystis* recurring, with one study finding that while it initially cleared the parasite it tended to reoccur at a higher rate six months later. And spontaneous clearance of the parasite was actually more common in the placebo group.[88]

There is the possibility that more natural treatment approaches could be effective, but these have not been well studied. A logical approach would be supporting the health of your gut bacteria with previously mentioned probiotics, prebiotics and dietary changes as it may be that *Blastocystis* is present because the dysbiosis associated with IBS allows it the opportunity to thrive. Indeed, a prevailing idea is that

Blastocystis is an opportunistic infection and a healthy gut environment would prevent it becoming a problem.

There are also a number of small clinical studies that have indicated certain natural medicines could be useful, including specific probiotics. One such study compared the therapeutic effect of the probiotic *Saccharomyces boulardii* to metronidazole and found that they had comparable effects for reduction of symptoms and elimination of the parasites.[89] The dose used in this study was 250 mg twice daily for fifteen days in children, with a typical dose for adults being 500 mg twice daily.

Herbal therapy also appears to be promising, with experimental studies showing a number of herbs with traditional use for digestive symptoms such as Black Cumin seed (*Nigella sativa*) and Chinese goldthread (*Coptis chinensis*), also have potential.[90,91] Interestingly, *Coptis chinensis* is rich in an anti-parasitic phytonutrient called Berberine which has been shown to relieve symptoms of IBS in a clinical study, but whether this was due to elimination of parasites was not tested.[92] The only clinical study of a herb, however, was on an emulsified oil of Oregano (*Origanum vulgare*) which appeared to be effective for some people at a dose of 200 mg three times daily for six weeks.[93] In addition to Oregano you could also try Berberine at a dose of 400 mg twice daily or Black Cumin seed capsules providing approximately 1000 mg of milled seeds twice daily for six weeks.[94]

Anti-candida program

Anti-candida therapy varies but often involves identification and elimination of food sensitivities, the restriction of refined sugars, nutritional supplementation that supports the immune system, natural antifungal treatments, and probiotics.[95] Some of the popular dietary approaches are extremely restrictive and unnecessary. For a simple and effective 'anti-candida program' try the following for 30 days in addition to the food plan on page 160.

Anti-candida 30-day program

1. Take an antimicrobial herbal formulation containing one or a combination of herbs such as Olive leaf (*Olea europaea*), Clove bud (*Syzygium aromaticum*), Oregano oil (*Origanum vulgare*), Barberry root (*Berberis vulgaris*), Thyme oil (*Thymus vulgaris*). Berberine HCl (500–1000 mg twice daily) or delayed-release Caprylic acid (400 mg 30 minutes before food three times daily) can also be effective. A typical dose is two capsules or tablets twice daily, but follow the manufacturer's recommendations.

2. Take a good probiotic once daily. This may help reduce the candida overgrowth and support healthy gut bacteria, which prevents the candida from returning. It is possible that certain probiotics would be more effective than others, but there is not yet enough research to recommend one probiotic over another for candida.

3. Take lactoferrin daily. Lactoferrin is a dietary supplement derived from dairy whey protein and has been shown to have important antimicrobial, antifungal and antiparasitic activity, with some evidence to show it could help reduce overgrowth of unfavourable micro-organisms such as candida

in the gut while promoting the growth of healthier bacteria.[96] A typical dose is 300 mg once daily.

Antibiotics

Some special types of antibiotics have been studied in IBS on the basis that they kill off bad gut bacteria and may therefore improve symptoms. The best studied of these is a drug called rifaximin, which is not absorbed into the bloodstream so it only works in the gut. Because it is not absorbed, the potential for rifaximin to cause side effects or allergic reactions is low.

Rifaximin appears to be generally effective for IBS, improving symptoms for up to several months after treatment in between 46 and 90 per cent of people. Rifaximin is typically used if there is evidence of SIBO (i.e. a positive hydrogen breath test) and has been shown to improve SIBO from 20 to 75 per cent of the time.[97] Treatment typically lasts from seven days to four weeks, depending on the dose, and is generally well tolerated. Less than 10 per cent of people experience side effects such as headache, nausea, diarrhoea and abdominal pain.[98]

There are problems with rifaximin, however. There is evidence that repeated, long-term use may cause antibiotic resistance, which limits its safety. Recent studies have shown that the benefits of rifaximin above placebo are a modest 10 to 15 per cent, and because research is preliminary it is not approved for use in IBS.[99,100]

So, as an alternative, you could try improving your gut flora with prebiotics and probiotics first, and if you have SIBO, try a twenty-day course of enteric-coated peppermint oil or one of the specific probiotics mentioned above. These approaches are more natural, safe and may work just as well.

TREATING THE CAUSE

Bad bacteria are usually present for a reason and even if you treat them with probiotics, prebiotics or peppermint oil, there is a chance the problem will just reoccur after time. The other chapters in this book address many of the reasons why you might have too many bad bugs and not enough good ones in your gastrointestinal tract, including chronic constipation, weak digestion, psychological stress, food intolerances (especially to gluten or lactose), too much dietary carbohydrate or a generally unhealthy diet. Making sure you address these reasons is key to improving your symptoms in the long term.

5

BOOST YOUR DIGESTION FOR BETTER HEALTH

After you chew and swallow food your digestive system secretes various digestive juices to help break down the food so you can absorb its nutrients. These major secretions are stomach acid, pancreatic enzymes and bile acids, and if production of any of these is low or their function is affected, it might lead to poorly digested food, bacterial overgrowth and subsequent problems that result in a wide range of digestive problems.

LOW STOMACH ACID

Chewing food in your mouth stimulates the taste buds, which signal to the digestive system to release digestive juices. Then as the food moves down your throat into your stomach, receptor cells sense it coming and trigger a major release of stomach acid. Digestion in the stomach involves the breakdown of large food pieces into smaller particles, which enables them to be easily digested and absorbed further down in the small intestine. Stomach acid also acts as an antibacterial shield, killing off potentially harmful germs from food and water, and protecting you from food-borne illness.

A reduction in stomach acid leads to subsequent poor digestion and the malabsorption of nutrients, and if you are not breaking down food efficiently you can develop food sensitivities as large protein molecules can remain intact and trigger a reaction in your immune system. Low stomach-acid production also reduces your natural antibacterial defences and can set you up for SIBO, an important underlying cause of digestive symptoms.

There is some evidence to suggest there may be a link between low stomach acid and common digestive problems. People with low stomach acid usually have symptoms that are similar to those of IBS, including indigestion, bloating or distention after meals, constipation, diarrhoea, excessive gas and chronic fatigue.

Symptoms that indicate low stomach acid may include:

- feeling unusually full after small or moderate-sized meals
- belching
- flatulence
- morning diarrhoea
- diarrhoea after heavy meals
- constipation
- heartburn
- indigestion
- a sensation that food sits for a long time in the stomach.[1]

A small clinical study in the 1960s found that giving people with low stomach acid betaine hydrochloride and pepsin, dietary supplements that help improve your stomach acid, relieved indigestion and excessive gas and reduced signs of inflammation in the gastrointestinal tract.[2] And an earlier study in the 1950s also suggested that supplementation with betaine hydrochloride could reduce bacterial overgrowth.[3] Unfortunately, since these very early studies, the possible link between low stomach acid and IBS has not been further explored.

The most common reasons for low stomach acid are increasing age, infection with the bacteria *Helicobacter pylori* and the use of antacid medications.[4] Chronic infection with *H. pylori* results in a condition known as atrophic gastritis, which causes inflammation in your stomach and a profound reduction in your gastric acid secretion. Infection with *H. pylori* is actually very common, with 20 per cent of people aged younger than 40 and 50 per cent of people aged over 60 affected. This increased likelihood of infection with age is the primary reason why older age is associated with lower stomach-acid production. However, even though atrophic gastritis is very common, most people don't know they have it because there are often no obvious symptoms, and it is not until a person undergoes a medical test for it that it is discovered.

It is difficult to know just how common *H. pylori* infection or atrophic gastritis is in IBS or whether it is a cause of symptoms, because it has not been well studied. However, some telling experimental studies have found that when you infect someone with *H. pylori* they suffer from pain, a constant feeling of fullness, nausea, vomiting, flatulence and fatigue, which are all characteristic symptoms of IBS. More evidence that *H. pylori* infection may be linked to IBS comes from a group of German researchers who observed that IBS sufferers with increased pain sensitivity were much more likely to be infected with *H. pylori*, suggesting that infection with this bacteria may indeed play an important role in IBS.[5]

Antacid medications are one of the most commonly used types of over-the-counter and prescription drugs. Because their purpose is either to neutralize or suppress your natural stomach acid production, and because they do this very effectively, they reduce your normal digestive function which, in turn, can lead to a host of problems including food sensitivities, nutritional imbalances, overgrowth of bad gut bacteria and, of course, IBS.[6] So, if you are using antacids regularly to get relief from heartburn, this could paradoxically be part of the reason you have a host of other symptoms.

LOW PANCREATIC ENZYMES

As food particles mixed with gastric acid exit your stomach they move into your small intestine where your pancreas is waiting to release pancreatic juice to further digest your food. Pancreatic juice is made up of bicarbonate and enzymes: the bicarbonate neutralizes the stomach acid so it does not corrode your intestines, and the enzymes are critical for the breakdown of protein, carbohydrate and fats.

A deficiency of pancreatic enzymes has not been classically thought to be a problem related to IBS but recent evidence suggests that, for some people, it could be a major reason for their symptoms.

A research group from the Department of Gastroenterology at Royal Hallamshire Hospital in Sheffield, England, decided to investigate for the first time whether people with IBS might have low pancreatic enzyme production.[7] What they found was that about 6 per cent of the people with IBS they tested had reduced pancreatic enzymes. This might not seem like many people but if you consider that IBS is thought to affect up to 30 per cent of the general population, low pancreatic enzyme production could be a cause of millions of cases of IBS, making this a very important discovery.

The research group then went on to prove something rather remarkable: they gave the people with low pancreatic enzyme production a dietary supplement of digestive enzymes and monitored any possible improvements in symptoms. Sure enough, after taking the digestive enzyme supplements, there were excellent improvements in IBS symptoms, in particular stool frequency, stool consistency and abdominal pain. The researchers also gave enzymes to people with IBS who did not have low pancreatic enzyme production and perhaps, not surprisingly, these people did not report any benefit.

So, how do you know if you have low pancreatic enzyme production? Well, your symptoms might give it away. Many people with IBS experience worse symptoms straight after eating, including bloating, pain and diarrhoea, which may actually indicate digestive enzyme deficiency. In fact, after hearing reports of excellent clinical benefits from a medical practice that was giving digestive enzymes to IBS patients before meals, a research group decided to formally test this theory with a study. They found that giving digestive enzyme supplements to people who reported diarrhoea, bloating and pain specifically after eating, was able to greatly improve their symptoms. The researchers even instructed people to eat meals that they knew triggered their symptoms, and the digestive enzymes still managed to work very well.[8]

If you find that your symptoms are particularly bad after a meal high in fats, a digestive enzyme supplement may be especially useful for you. Taking digestive enzymes has been clearly shown to reduce bloating, gas and feelings of fullness after a high-fat meal.[9] And for people with IBS, digestive enzyme supplementation can help improve fat digestion and reduce symptoms of intolerance to dietary fats too.[10]

Why exactly some people with IBS might have low pancreatic enzyme production is not yet clear. Two possible causes that need to be investigated are gluten sensitivity and a condition known as chronic pancreatitis. Chronic pancreatitis usually presents with severe attacks of abdominal pain and may be related to heavy alcohol use over decades.[11] Chronic pancreatitis is, however, quite rare, with about 1 in 10,000 thought to have the condition. Gluten sensitivity on the other hand is not uncommon, affecting approximately 1 in 100, and is even more common in people with IBS. Gluten sensitivity is a topic we will cover in more detail later.

BILE ACID DIARRHOEA

Along with stomach acid and pancreatic enzymes, the third major type of digestive juice is bile acids. Bile acids or bile salts are produced by your liver and secreted into your small intestine by your gall bladder in response to eating a meal containing fats, which would normally be most meals.

The major function of bile salts is to help you absorb dietary fats and they do this by binding with the fats and carrying them into your bloodstream in a process known as emulsification. Most of the bile salts secreted by your liver are used to carry fats into your blood, which are then recycled back through the liver with very little, less than 5 per cent, excreted in your stools. So, put simply, bile salts help you digest and absorb fat and are then reused again and again.

If this normal process of bile salt recycling is disrupted, you end up with unusually high amounts of the bile salts passing through your gut, and you can start to develop problems. When large amounts of bile salts reach your large intestine, they can dramatically increase the passage of water into your colon, which can lead to diarrhoea and related symptoms such as bloating, urgency and faecal incontinence.[12] Bile acid malabsorption and the subsequent digestive problems that arise are known as bile acid diarrhoea.

Bile acid diarrhoea has only been investigated recently as a possible cause of IBS, and it turns out it is a major issue for a lot of people. A research group from the Department of Nutrition and Dietetics at the Royal Marsden Hospital in England conducted an analysis of eighteen studies to see just how common bile acid diarrhoea is in IBS sufferers.[13] What they found was that up to 30 per cent of IBS sufferers with diarrhoea-predominant symptoms (IBS-D) had some degree of bile acid diarrhoea, making it a remarkably common problem, and certainly much more common than previously thought.

Professor Julian Walters from the Imperial College London, who was involved in this research, has suggested that a possible cause of bile acid diarrhoea is an overproduction of bile acids due to an inability of the body to realize it is already producing enough. In support of this theory, people with bile acid diarrhoea tend to have lower levels of a hormone produced in the small intestine that lets the liver know enough bile acids have been produced and to hold back on production until the next meal.[14] But why would you get stuck in this state of overproduction in the first place?

Interestingly, the development of bile acid diarrhoea may be due to other known causes of IBS including parasitic infection, SIBO and low pancreatic enzyme production. While bile acid diarrhoea is typically managed with medication, treating bacterial overgrowth and supplementing with digestive enzymes has also been shown to improve the condition.[15] To decipher whether you have bile acid diarrhoea, trial a course of digestive enzymes first and if they do not improve things you may need to investigate whether you have SIBO. As a last resort speak to your doctor about bile acid binder medication.

IS WEAK DIGESTION A CAUSE OF YOUR SYMPTOMS?

There are a few things you need to consider to help find out if weak digestion is causing your symptoms:

Does eating make symptoms worse? Most people report that their symptoms are worse after eating and, although this is not a definitive sign that your problem is related to weak digestion, it may indicate that low stomach acid, low pancreatic enzymes or bile acid diarrhoea are to blame, especially if you notice fatty meals or certain foods are a trigger.

Test for atrophic gastritis: Next to antacid medications the most common cause of low stomach acid is chronic atrophic gastritis. You need to speak to your healthcare professional about testing for atrophic gastritis because they can advise you on whether or not testing is necessary. Furthermore, testing is complicated and may require a number of different tests. A blood test for *H. pylori* is an accurate way to identify infection, but other tests like an endoscopy may be required.

Test for low pancreatic enzymes: Testing your levels of faecal elastase 1 (a type of pancreatic enzyme) is a very accurate way of finding out whether or not your pancreatic enzyme production is low. A level higher than 200 mcg per gram is considered normal, while lower than 100 clearly indicates low enzyme production. Detection of mild enzyme deficiency, which would be somewhere between 100 and 200, is much less accurate, but a number between these two figures may indicate low enzymes are a problem. The test involves providing a stool sample. You could also just try taking digestive enzymes with meals to see if your symptoms improve because this test is not always accurate.

Test for bile acid diarrhoea: The SeHCAT (Se-homocholic acid taurine) test is the best way to assess whether or not you have bile acid diarrhoea, however the test it is not available in many countries and even if it is, it is not commonly used. Nonetheless, the SeHCAT test is a safe and relatively low-cost way to identify whether or not you have bile acid diarrhoea. Another way to test for bile acid diarrhoea is to trial a bile acid binder medication, which is used to treat bile acid diarrhoea, and if you respond to treatment it is a reasonable indicator that bile acid diarrhoea is a major problem. You will need to speak to a licensed healthcare professional about the suitability of medication.

HOW TO IMPROVE YOUR DIGESTION

Betaine hydrochloride

Taking a betaine hydrochloride supplement is a simple and effective way to increase your stomach acid (hydrochloric acid). Often pepsin is added to the supplement but there is no evidence to suggest it would have any additional benefit. It is important to note that this treatment has not been proven to relieve IBS, but a number of studies have shown that it can increase your stomach acid and improve related symptoms such as indigestion, bloating, constipation, diarrhoea, excessive gas and fatigue, so it's certainly worth trying.

Try taking one capsule containing 650 mg of betaine hydrochloride with each meal. One capsule might be enough to improve your symptoms but, if not, you may need to increase the dose slowly by one capsule per meal up to a maximum of three capsules per meal. You can use fewer capsules with smaller meals and more capsules with larger meals.[16,17]

Betaine hydrochloride is very safe, however you should not use this treatment if you are also regularly taking non-steroidal anti-inflammatory medications (e.g. aspirin, ibuprofen, paracetamol) or corticosteroids. Also, do not take betaine hydrochloride if you have an existing peptic ulcer or upper abdominal pain. And if you experience abdominal pain or burning, stop taking it immediately and seek medical advice if the pain persists.

Herbal bitters

Herbal bitters have a long traditional history of use for indigestion and are still used widely in many parts of the world, where they are often taken after meals as a 'digestive'. One such herb that is particularly popular is the roots of Gentian (*Gentiana lutea*), a yellow flowering plant commonly found in the mountain regions of central and south Europe. Gentian contains bitter substances which have been shown to stimulate the secretion of saliva in the mouth, as well as hydrochloric acid in the stomach.[18,19]

In one study, people with various symptoms including heartburn, vomiting, stomach aches, nausea, loss of appetite, constipation and flatulence were treated with capsules containing 120 mg of Gentian root extract two to three times daily for fifteen days. Improvements in symptoms were evident after five days in most cases, and by the end of the study the average level of improvement was 68 per cent. The efficacy of the preparation was assessed by the doctors as excellent (symptoms eliminated) in 31 per cent of patients, good in a further 55 per cent, moderate in 9 per cent and inadequate in only 5 per cent of cases.[20] So as an alternative or complement to betaine hydrochloride you could also try Gentian root or some old-fashioned herbal bitters with heavy meals.

Digestive enzymes

Digestive enzyme supplements have been shown to improve IBS symptoms, especially in people in whom testing has revealed low pancreatic enzyme production or in those who experience worse symptoms after eating.

There are a remarkable number of dietary enzyme supplements available on the market with many different ingredients at many different dosages, making it hard to work out which is best. To make it simple, you need to find a product that preferably contains at least the enzymes lipase (digests fats), protease (digests protein) and amylase (digests carbohydrate). These are available as standard animal-derived or vegetarian enzymes.

The lipase content is the best reference for determining how strong the product is and according to clinical studies needs to be at a dose of about 8000–24,000 USP (United States Pharmacopeia) units of lipase per meal for animal-derived products, which are also commonly labelled as 'pancreatin derived enzymes'.[21] However, the units used to measure enzymes can vary a lot and be hard to interpret, so alternatively you can look at the total milligram (mg) amount of enzymes in the capsule — a good potency would be around 400 mg total enzymes per capsule.

There is evidence to suggest that vegetarian enzymes (from sources such as the fungus *Aspergillus*) may be a better option. Apart from the fact that the source is more ethical, they are more stable and resistant to stomach acid, and may actually work better as a result.[22] The way vegetarian enzymes are measured is not consistent and the dose and potency of these products varies considerably. So, if you are using vegetarian enzymes make sure the product contains the enzymes lipase, protease and amylase and follow the dosage recommendations on the product label, which is typically one to two capsules per meal.

Generally, digestive enzymes do not have any side effects, apart from perhaps transient gastrointestinal upset or nausea, and you should experience beneficial effects relatively quickly, sometimes within a single meal. Even if you don't notice an immediate benefit, you should continue to use the enzymes as studies have shown the optimal therapeutic effects occur after about three months. After a while you might want to use digestive enzymes only with meals you know can trigger your symptoms.

Avoid alpha-glucosidase inhibitors

Alpha-glucosidase is an enzyme in your digestive system that helps break down and digest carbohydrates. A number of natural foods have been shown to inhibit the action of alpha-glucosidase and some pharmaceutical drugs have been specifically developed to do this.

Because they prevent the digestion of carbohydrate, alpha-glucosidase inhibitor drugs are used for diabetes and obesity, the rationale being that if you block the breakdown of carbohydrates you absorb fewer calories as sugars. However, interfering with the digestion of carbohydrates can cause problems and common side effects of these medications are flatulence, diarrhoea and abdominal pain.

Many natural foods are also alpha-glucosidase inhibitors, especially foods commonly reported as IBS triggers — spicy foods, beans, onions, garlic, corn and chillies. The dietary supplements white kidney bean and mulberry leaf are alpha-glucosidase inhibitors too. You may find that avoiding these foods, or taking a digestive enzyme supplement when you consume these foods, will help improve your digestion and reduce symptoms.[23]

Try a low bile acid diet

Apart from using digestive enzymes or bile acid binder medications, or by addressing the symptoms of SIBO, people with bile acid diarrhoea can also improve with dietary changes.

Avoiding high-fat meals is a standard recommendation and can reduce the risk of diarrhoea.[24-26] In addition, avoiding meals that contain lots of refined sugars might make a difference as sugar, like fat, can stimulate bile acid production.[27]

Eating more natural fibre from wholegrains, fruits and vegetables has been shown to decrease bile acids and could be helpful.[28,29] One study found that eating sun-dried raisins (about 85 g a day) could reduce bile acid excretion and improve regularity.[30]

6

CLEAR CONSTIPATION AND REBOOT YOUR SYSTEM

Chronic constipation is a very common feature of IBS and although typically considered a symptom, there is good reason to believe that for some people it may actually be the underlying cause of the most troubling complaints, including bloating, discomfort, pain and even occasional diarrhoea.

In medical terms, the diagnosis of IBS is separated from chronic constipation by the presence of pain so, by strict definition, if you have constipation with pain, you have IBS, according to the textbooks at least. This means that the idea that constipation could actually cause IBS has not been given much attention.[1]

Over ten years ago, Professor John Hunter and his colleagues from the gastroenterology unit at Addenbrooke's Hospital in the United Kingdom discovered that a number of their IBS patients suffered from what they called 'overload and overflow' syndrome. As the name suggests, what they found was that constipation can build up a backlog or 'overload' of faecal matter that eventually reaches a critical threshold or tipping point, which then causes diarrhoea or 'overflow'. The overflow or diarrhoea tended to happen intermittently, about every seven to fourteen days.

They found that giving these patients a 'bowel clear-out' with a strong laxative, similar to the protocol used before colonoscopy, was able to remove the backlog of constipation and get things moving again, much like clearing out a blocked drainpipe. They then had their patients follow the initial clear-out with a daily flaxseed (linseed) fibre supplement, which acts as a bulking laxative to keep things regular. This regime was incredibly successful for the people with 'overload and overflow' and in a clinical study was able to completely eliminate symptoms of IBS in the majority of people with this problem for at least six months.[2]

Importantly, the people treated by Professor John Hunter's group did not realize they were constipated because they tended to have a bowel motion most days, but as it turned out, the stools they were passing were Types 1 and 2 on the Bristol Stool Scale (see page 26), which is a better indicator of poor transit time and constipation regardless of how frequently you go to the toilet. Remember that bowel movements ranging from three times daily to three times a week are considered normal, so frequency is an unreliable indicator of constipation.

Recent research provides support for Professor Hunter's early pioneering observation that clearing constipation can be an effective way to treat digestive symptoms. Radio imaging studies of the gastrointestinal tract have since revealed that many people with IBS symptoms have 'hidden constipation', which is the build-up of faeces in the large bowel regardless of whether or not they have daily bowel motions. This build-up means you can have an unusually high level of faecal matter in your bowel placing pressure against your bowel wall, causing distention and in turn bloating, discomfort and pain.[3] IBS sufferers tend to have a highly sensitive gut and any increase in pressure against the gut wall is going to cause problems. It has also been found that treating people who have hidden constipation with drugs that improve elimination can greatly reduce symptoms and improve quality of life.[4]

And it turns out that constipation can, indeed, cause diarrhoea, which goes against conventional wisdom that you mostly have either one problem or the other. In fact, chronic constipation and the build-up of compacted faeces has long been associated with diarrhoea and faecal incontinence outside of IBS research and especially in the elderly. This is because a backlog of faeces can cause newer faecal matter to liquefy as it passes the blockage and then travels through the gut as diarrhoea. Compacted faeces may also irritate the gut, causing increased production of mucus and further contributing to diarrhoea.[5]

Professor Hunter and his group found that not all their patients had compacted faecal matter; rather, their theory for the constipation–diarrhoea connection is that constipation builds up to a critical mass at which point common triggers, such as a rich meal or stress, cause the build-up to be rapidly expelled in a burst of pain and diarrhoea. So, in summary, whether due to compacted faeces or a constipated backlog, it is possible for constipation to cause a wide range of digestive symptoms. Further, constipation may cause intermittent bouts of diarrhoea, explaining why diarrhoea may be present even though constipation is the cause of your overall symptoms.

CAUSES OF CONSTIPATION

For years the cause of chronic constipation has been attributed to simple diet and lifestyle factors such as lack of regular exercise, not eating enough fibre or drinking enough water, but simply addressing these does not always improve constipation. For example, less than 30 per cent of people with constipation improve after increasing their fibre intake and, in fact, increasing fibre can sometimes make symptoms, such as bloating and pain, a lot worse. The disappointing effects of these standard diet and lifestyle recommendations for constipation indicate there are other possible reasons for a sluggish bowel.[6]

Changes in your gut bacteria may help explain why some people develop constipation. We know that IBS sufferers tend to have important differences in their gut bacteria, namely more bad bugs, fewer good bifidobacteria and sometimes small intestinal bacterial overgrowth (SIBO). People with chronic constipation tend to have similar issues in their gut bacteria and this might directly explain why they are constipated. Your gut bacteria are able to influence the muscular contractions of your gut and the total gut transit time, so any disturbances in your gut bacteria could certainly cause constipation by fundamentally changing your gut function. In support of this theory, some probiotic supplements have been shown to improve gut transit time and help relieve constipation.[7]

Your ability to pass a normal stool is also influenced by a series of voluntary muscles including your abdominal muscles, pelvic floor muscles and anal sphincter. An inability to relax these muscles or an increase in contractions of the anal sphincter results in difficulty defecating and is a common cause of chronic constipation.[8] Perhaps not surprisingly, many IBS sufferers often have difficulty with these muscles, which is medically known as a defecatory disorder.[9] People with defecatory disorder as a cause of their constipation tend not to get any better with laxatives or a high-fibre diet and may even have bad reactions to them. Fortunately, there is not actually a problem with the muscles themselves, it's just that they require training so they contract properly. Treatment with biofeedback therapy can help re-educate the muscles so they contract properly, and is very effective for eliminating defecatory disorder and improving bowel regularity.[10]

Because of the close connection between the gut and your central nervous system, known as the gut–brain axis (see page 137), chronic stress may also play a role in the development of constipation. Most people with IBS can link stress to their symptoms in some way and constipation has been linked to changes in nervous-system function.[11] There is some evidence to show that managing stress more effectively with mind–body therapies can help with relaxation and improve many digestive symptoms, including constipation.[12]

Food intolerances are also an important but underappreciated and often completely neglected cause of constipation. For example, one study found that women with constipation who had failed to improve with increased fibre intake or laxatives were able to successfully eliminate constipation by the identification and removal of problematic foods.[13] Interestingly, foods that caused the constipation were not only common problem foods such as wheat, cow's milk and eggs but also less obvious ones such as tomato, beef and cauliflower. So foods you think are healthy could be actually causing your problems. Food intolerances can activate your immune system, cause inflammation and adversely affect the normal function of the muscles in your gut involved in the passage of food, thus explaining the link to constipation.[14]

So as you can see, the standard recommendations of exercise, fibre and water are only a small part of the bigger picture. Healthy and regular elimination also depends on good gut bacteria, proper relaxation and contraction of your abdominal and pelvic floor muscles, stress management and the identification of problem foods. In many cases, clearing out any build-up with a strong laxative regime may also be necessary. If these are not addressed, fibre and general laxative use tends to just make things worse.

HOW DO YOU KNOW IF CONSTIPATION IS A PROBLEM?

Firstly, use the Bristol Stool Scale (see page 26) to determine whether you suffer from constipation. Constipation may seem easy to identify but many people who are constipated don't know it. This is because people tend to associate constipation with straining, hard stools, time spent on the toilet, a sense of incomplete evacuation or not having a bowel movement for a few days. However, you could have these symptoms yet not actually be constipated. The best way to check is to use the Bristol Stool Scale. If you are regularly passing stools that fall into the Type 1 or Type 2 categories you are constipated, even if you are going regularly or have occasional diarrhoea.

WHAT CAN YOU DO TO TREAT CONSTIPATION?

There are several options you can try to treat chronic constipation and relieve your digestive complaints, including a constipation clear-out, a digestive kick-start and biofeedback therapy. These are much more likely to produce better and longer-lasting results than laxative use and may help completely resolve your symptoms.

Kick-start your digestive system

In his excellent book *Irritable Bowel Solutions: The essential guide to IBS, its causes and treatments*, Dr John Hunter describes a protocol he has successfully used for clearing out constipation completely. He suggests this as a starting point for treating chronic constipation.

The idea is to firstly clear out your bowels with a strong laxative and subsequently encourage regular and complete evacuation with ground flaxseeds (linseeds), which act as a bulk-forming laxative. Ground or milled flaxseeds are used because they do not ferment to create gas and are thus much better tolerated than other types of fibre, especially in people with IBS.

Because the protocol Dr Hunter developed uses a very strong laxative that has occasional side effects, a slower and more natural approach based on new research into a surprising fruit for digestive health may be a better alternative — restarting your digestive system using the humble kiwifruit.

For some years kiwifruit had been anecdotally reported to have a gentle laxative effect, so a research group from the Auckland University of Technology in New Zealand conducted a study with older-age adults giving them two to three kiwifruit a day for a few weeks. They found that eating kiwifruit led to a bulkier and softer stool, as well as more frequent bowel movements.[15]

A number of subsequent studies in people suffering from constipation have also found that eating kiwifruit daily for about four weeks relieves constipation, improves bowel transit time, results in better shaped stools (on the Bristol Stool Scale), reduces bloating, improves general comfort and satisfaction and decreases laxative use. And eating kiwifruit has been shown to relieve constipation and overall digestive symptoms in IBS sufferers as well.[16–18]

Kiwifruit is turning out to be quite the digestive health superfood; its proven benefits for relieving constipation and improving digestive health are most likely due to the fact that it is unusually high in digestive enzymes, prebiotics and a unique gentle fibre that swells after digestion and improves bowel movements. In fact, research has shown kiwifruit can help digest protein, increase good bacteria and improve gastric emptying.[19-21]

Kiwifruit kick-start instructions

1. Each morning for breakfast consume two to three 'green fuzzy' kiwifruit (*Actinidia deliciosa*), not the smooth yellow variety. You could also take a single 2.5–5 g dose of a kiwifruit dietary supplement standardized to the enzyme actinidin, as this can also work well.

2. Shortly after consuming the kiwifruit drink two glasses (500 ml) of water.

3. Continue your daily kiwifruit or kiwifruit supplement for four weeks.

4. During the initial four weeks do not take any fibre supplements and avoid foods with added fibre such as cereals and cereal grain products.

5. The kiwifruit should slowly improve your bowel movements, reduce bloating and leave you feeling much more comfortable over the coming weeks.

6. After the four weeks you can stop the kiwifruit and start taking 1 tablespoon of ground flaxseeds

(linseeds) instead. This is easily sprinkled onto cereals, food or simply mixed in water and drunk. Follow with two glasses of water.

7. You can increase the dose up to 2 tablespoons of flaxseeds twice daily, but you may need only 1 tablespoon daily as too much could cause bloating and discomfort. Remember to follow with two glasses of water. Once you have found the right dosage for you, you should pass regular stools and prevent constipation again.

8. You should not need to repeat the program, but if you do find the effects wearing off, stop the flaxseeds and try consuming kiwifruit daily again until your symptoms improve.

If you can't obtain kiwifruit easily, you could use papaya (*Carica papaya*) instead. Papaya is rich in a digestive enzyme called papain and, like kiwifruit, has also been shown in a number of studies to relieve constipation and improve digestive symptoms.[22] Simply consume about 2 cups of chopped fresh papaya, or 20–40 ml of a papaya paste supplement, in place of the kiwifruit.

Take ground flaxseeds regularly

Flaxseeds (linseeds) are a popular treatment for the symptoms of constipation, bloating and flatulence and have been included in a number of professional recommendations for IBS treatment.[23] Studies have shown that taking flaxseeds regularly can improve bowel regularity and, unlike other types of fibre, flaxseeds do not tend to ferment, produce gas and make symptoms worse.

In a study of people with constipation-predominant IBS (IBS-C), taking ground flaxseeds (linseeds) daily for three months significantly reduced constipation, bloating and discomfort and people continued to benefit while continuing to take flaxseeds months later.[24] Start with a heaped teaspoon of ground flaxseeds twice daily with meals and follow with a glass of water. You can slowly increase the dose up to 2 tablespoons twice daily if you find you need to.

Probiotics

Some probiotics have been shown to help reduce symptoms of constipation and improve regularity, including in people with IBS. Probiotics can also help to reduce other symptoms such as pain and bloating. The reason probiotics are thought to be useful is due to their ability to improve the balance of gut bacteria, reducing bacterial species that could be directly responsible for constipation and increasing those that improve gastrointestinal health.[25] A review of fourteen probiotic studies found that as a whole, probiotics significantly reduced whole gut transit time by 12.4 hours and improved stool frequency; however, some probiotics were found to be more effective than others.[26] Probiotics that have been shown in good clinical studies to be particularly promising for improving regularity include *Bifidobacterium lactis* HN019, VSL#3, *Lactobacillus reuteri* DSM 17938, and Bifidobacteria species in general, although it is not yet clear exactly which probiotics are the best and it is likely a different product could work better for you.[27-30]

Prunes

An ancient remedy for constipation, dried plums, commonly known as prunes, have been used for over a thousand years. The great Iranian physician Avicenna (980–1037 CE) reportedly proposed that prunes provide a slippery surface to facilitate movement, which may well be right — modern research suggests prunes gently stimulate gastrointestinal secretion and muscular function.[31] Although prunes may promote regularity due to their sorbitol content, and sorbitol is known to aggravate symptoms in people with IBS, prunes may have a more complex reason for their benefits, including their content of phytonutrients, and based on clinical experience they are very unlikely to make symptoms worse.[32] In one study of people with chronic constipation, 100 grams a day of prunes for three weeks improved stool frequency and stool consistency and was more effective than psyllium fibre.[33] Thus you could try 100 grams, or about nine prunes, daily for three weeks as a natural approach to restoring regularity.

Biofeedback therapy

Biofeedback therapy has been shown to be very effective for people who have a defecatory disorder or constipation, due to problems relaxing the muscles that allow for healthy bowel movement. You will first need to be assessed for whether or not you have a defecatory disorder, typically using a defecography examination, so it is best to speak to your doctor or gastroenterologist to see if you require testing. Therapy involves retraining your muscles by directly measuring their function while you receive visual and/or auditory feedback. This treatment has a good success rate, with about 67 per cent of people experiencing long-lasting benefits.[34]

Treat the underlying cause

There are a number of potential causes of chronic constipation addressed in the other chapters of this book including food intolerances, coeliac disease, weak digestion, chronic psychological stress and bacterial overgrowth. If you are going to improve constipation and your digestive health in the long term, you may find you need to address one or a number of these factors, otherwise you may end up dependent on laxatives, which is not ideal.

7

UNCOVER SECRET PROBLEM FOODS

Over 60 per cent of people with IBS report that their symptoms get worse after eating, with 93 per cent experiencing problems within three hours of a meal, especially when consuming foods rich in carbohydrates and fat, coffee, alcohol and hot spices.[1] Classic symptoms such as bloating, pain and diarrhoea often occur after eating and because of this many people with digestive symptoms believe they have food intolerances, but it is important to remember that eating food is the most powerful trigger of gastrointestinal function there is, and just because eating makes things worse, it does not always mean food intolerances are the problem.

Before questioning the role of food intolerance, consider that the gastrointestinal system in IBS sufferers is in a unique state of dysfunction, so it should be no surprise that simply eating can trigger symptoms. Food is a complex mixture of constituents such as fibre, nutrients, fat and thousands of naturally occurring chemicals and as it passes through an inflamed, hypersensitive gut it is going to be likely to cause unpredictable problems. Studies have found, for example, that pain and discomfort can be exaggerated by fatty meals because too much fat heightens pain sensitivity, and it is possible that simply overeating could cause increased pressure against your gut wall, leading to distention and feelings of bloating and pain.[2]

There is also a psychosomatic component to food intolerance to be mindful of before jumping to conclusions. Simply thinking a kind of food makes your symptoms worse can be enough for the food to trigger symptoms. In fact, up to 75 per cent of people who report having food intolerance don't react to the foods when they eat them unknowingly.[3] So it is important not to mistakenly assume that foods are always a problem as this can lead to unnecessary restrictive eating, which can make things worse, as well as create a great deal of anxiety and stress. However, many people with IBS *do* have real food intolerances and clinical studies have shown that eliminating problem foods can lead to dramatic improvements in symptoms and sometimes complete relief. The most common food intolerances are caused by gluten-containing grains and dairy products.

GLUTEN-CONTAINING GRAINS

While cereal grains such as wholegrain rye and wheat may appear healthy, for some people they can be the cause of IBS symptoms and eliminating gluten from your diet can result in a complete recovery.

Gluten is a protein found in wheat, barley and rye that, when poorly digested, can cause an autoimmune disease in genetically susceptible individuals — this is known as coeliac disease, a severe form of food intolerance. If you have coeliac disease and eat gluten, your immune system strongly reacts to the gluten in your digestive system and damages the lining of your small intestine. While coeliac disease was traditionally thought to be a rare problem and limited to the digestive tract, it is now known to be remarkably common and has been linked to a wide range of seemingly unrelated symptoms beyond the digestive system.[4]

Classic digestive symptoms of coeliac disease include abdominal pain or discomfort, constipation, diarrhoea and bloating, so you can see why undiagnosed gluten intolerance may be an issue. Other symptoms of coeliac disease that are common in IBS are anxiety, depression and chronic fatigue. And there are many other symptoms that can be linked to gluten intolerance, such as weight loss, tingling numbness in the hands and feet, migraine headaches, a rash known as dermatitis herpetiformis, autoimmune diseases and thyroid disease.[5] These additional symptoms may or may not be present but if you have any of them they can help reveal whether gluten is the problem.

Symptoms associated with coeliac disease[6-8]

Age group	Associated symptoms and illnesses
Infants	Diarrhoea, abdominal distention, failure to thrive, vomiting, irritability, anorexia and constipation.
Children	Short stature, behavioural problems, learning disabilities, skin problems and anaemia.
Adults	Chronic unexplained diarrhoea, which may be accompanied by abdominal pain or discomfort. Constipation, bloating, iron-deficiency anaemia, osteoporosis, weight loss, depression or anxiety, tingling numbness in the hands and feet, recurrent migraine, a rash known as dermatitis herpetiformis, irritable bowel syndrome, autoimmune disorders, thyroid disease and chronic fatigue.

The prevalence of coeliac disease in the general population is quite common, affecting approximately one in 100 people, and it is considerably higher in people who have relatives with coeliac disease.[9] A large-scale analysis of some fourteen studies found that coeliac disease was four times more common in people with IBS than in the general public.[10] Because of the very high frequency of coeliac disease in IBS, routine blood testing is now recommended whenever someone is diagnosed with IBS, especially for people with diarrhoea as a major symptom.[11] But, unfortunately, coeliac disease is still poorly recognized by medical professionals, and sufferers generally report symptoms for eleven to twelve years before a diagnosis, even though they may seek help. People with coeliac disease also generally receive one or more wrong diagnoses before coeliac disease is properly identified.[12]

For many years a number of people have noticed that their symptoms got better by following a gluten-free diet, even though tests came back negative for coeliac disease. Research has now clearly demonstrated that people can have gluten intolerance without coeliac disease, which means even though a blood or other diagnostic test may come back negative, you may still have what is referred to as non-coeliac gluten sensitivity.

Although many people instinctively know they are sensitive to gluten yet do not have coeliac disease, until recently non-coeliac gluten sensitivity had not been well studied. To try to shed light on the matter a research group from Monash University in Australia decided to study a group of people with IBS who did not have any evidence of coeliac disease, to see if their symptoms changed on a gluten-containing or a gluten-free diet. Sure enough, those on a gluten-containing diet had much worse symptoms than those on a gluten-free diet, and those who went gluten free had improvements in overall symptoms, especially with pain, bloating, stool consistency and tiredness.[13] This discovery suggests that non-coeliac gluten sensitivity is indeed very real and can cause IBS symptoms.

Importantly, the researchers could not find any biological reason why people in the study were intolerant to gluten; even with a suite of tests looking at changes in their immune and gastrointestinal systems, everything seemed to be normal. Though this may make non-coeliac gluten sensitivity look like an enigma, it simply means we do not yet understand how it occurs and, importantly, this also explains why tests don't always reliably detect gluten intolerance.

If you have coeliac disease or a gluten sensitivity, going gluten-free can have a life-changing effect. In one of the earliest studies of a gluten-free diet, 105 people with IBS were tested for coeliac disease and then put on a gluten-free diet for six months. Twelve people (11.4 per cent) were discovered to have coeliac disease and eleven of these stuck to the diet. Subsequently all of them had major improvements in their symptoms and three no longer had any symptoms at all after the six months.[14] Since this study a number of much larger investigations have shown that most people with digestive symptoms who are diagnosed with coeliac disease and start a gluten-free diet experience substantial benefit or complete resolution of their symptoms.[15]

DAIRY PRODUCTS

Along with gluten-containing grains, dairy products are among the most common sources of food intolerance for IBS sufferers. There are two general reasons why dairy products might lead to IBS symptoms: firstly, they often contain lactose and lactose intolerance can cause digestive problems; and secondly, other components of dairy products such as fats, proteins or chemicals that are broken down during digestion could be triggering symptoms.

Lactose is a sugar that naturally occurs in dairy foods and is often added as a sweetener to many other foods such as soft drinks or sodas. The problem of lactose intolerance arises when you have low levels of the digestive enzyme lactase in your small intestine and you are unable to sufficiently break down and digest lactose. Undigested lactose in your digestive system can ferment and release toxic byproducts that cause symptoms such as abdominal discomfort, bloating, wind and diarrhoea.[16]

We are all born with high levels of lactase to help digest our mother's milk, but the levels gradually decline with age. If your lactase levels drop low enough, you can end up with lactose intolerance, which incidentally is less common in cultural groups that have been consuming dairy foods for longer. Only about 2 to 22 per cent of Europeans are lactose intolerant because of a long history of consuming dairy foods, but as many as 60 to 100 per cent of people with Asian and African ancestry, for whom dairy foods are relatively new, cannot sufficiently digest lactose.[17]

If you are lactose intolerant there is a wide range of symptoms that can occur if you consume too much lactose, some of which may be surprising as they are not simply digestive problems:

- abdominal pain
- distention and bloating
- stomach growling, rumbling or gurgling
- flatulence
- diarrhoea
- constipation
- nausea

- vomiting
- headache and light-headedness
- loss of concentration and poor short-term memory
- long-term severe tiredness or fatigue
- muscle pain
- joint pain, and/or swelling and stiffness
- allergies (eczema, itching, rhinitis, sinusitis)
- mouth ulcers
- acne
- depression.[18,19]

These symptoms vary considerably from person to person and may occur hours or even several days after lactose consumption, making it difficult to connect your symptoms to lactose. However, diarrhoea does tend to be more common in people who have lactose intolerance, so if diarrhoea is a predominant symptom, you definitely need to rule out the possibility of lactose intolerance.[20]

Often people do not associate lactose or dairy products with their symptoms and there are a few reasons for this: people with lactose intolerance can safely consume up to 6 g of lactose (equivalent to about a quarter of a glass of milk) in a single serving without any symptoms.[21] So small amounts are generally tolerated but more than this can start to cause problems. And some dairy foods contain very little or no lactose, such as natural yoghurt and hard cheeses. Also, symptoms can be delayed by up to a week after eating lactose, so it can be difficult to link them to the problem foods. And finally, lactose is used as an additive in many common and surprising foods, such as processed meats, bread, soft drinks and beer, and often is not listed on the product label, so you could still have symptoms of lactose intolerance even though you think you are avoiding dairy foods.[22]

It's quite clear that a number of people with digestive problems may actually have undiagnosed lactose intolerance and, what's more, avoiding lactose can in some cases resolve all of their symptoms.

A study of 230 people with suspected IBS found that lactose malabsorption was relatively common; in fact, 157 patients (68.2 per cent) were diagnosed with lactose intolerance. Once lactose intolerance was identified, 110 of the IBS sufferers went on a lactose-free diet. Of those who followed the diet, 43.6 per cent eliminated their symptoms completely; however, for some people, symptoms were only modestly reduced, and in a smaller percentage symptoms did not change at all.[23]

Another study found that in a group of 70 IBS sufferers 24.3 per cent had lactose intolerance. They then started a lactose-free diet and had their symptoms assessed some five years later. Of those who stuck to the diet, 87.5 per cent no longer had any symptoms and had collectively dropped their medical visits by 75 per cent.[24]

Beyond lactose intolerance it is possible that dairy foods are problematic because they are causing an allergic or hypersensitivity reaction. While true dairy-food allergy is very rare in adults, it is possible to have what is known as a delayed hypersensitivity reaction. This is a type of reaction that cannot be detected with classic allergy testing and can develop insidiously after eating the offending food, from as little as one hour and up to seven days, which is why it is called 'delayed hypersensitivity'. Like lactose intolerance, gastrointestinal symptoms commonly include nausea, bloating, discomfort and diarrhoea.[25]

There is a wide range of possible substances in dairy foods that could be linked to a delayed hypersensitivity reaction, in particular dairy proteins (such as casein). So, in some cases, dairy foods may be best avoided completely.

OTHER PROBLEM FOODS

For some people a number of different food intolerances could be causing digestive symptoms. Identifying exactly which foods are causing problems can be difficult and time consuming but ultimately rewarding. There are two ways to identify food intolerances that have been shown to work relatively well: an elimination and re-challenge diet, which involves following, for a few weeks, an introductory diet only of foods unlikely to cause symptoms and then adding back suspect foods every one to four days and seeing if you react to them; or testing for specific immune markers called immunoglobulin G (IgG) that can help identify potential problem foods. If you have high IgG markers to a particular food, then it might be triggering symptoms. Using both methods to identify problem foods and then eliminating them from your diet has been shown to be very helpful.

Several studies assessing the efficacy of elimination and re-challenge diets with IBS sufferers found that positive responses from these diets vary from about 5 to 71 per cent. The most common problem foods were found to be milk, wheat, coffee and eggs but also included tea, nuts, peas, citrus fruits, yeast, onions, butter, chocolate and cheese.[26] Unfortunately, all of these studies were conducted over twenty years ago and their methods and accuracy have been questioned. The wide variation in how much people benefit from elimination and re-challenge diets certainly throws some doubt on just how beneficial the approach is. Nevertheless, an elimination and re-challenge diet is perhaps the most accurate way to identify problem foods and may be very helpful for improving your symptoms, but because it is quite restrictive, it should be embarked upon under the supervision of a qualified nutrition professional.

The use of IgG testing has more recently shown some promise and is certainly a less painstaking and much faster method of identifying problem foods. The first study to examine the potential benefits of dietary elimination based on IgG testing found that this approach resulted in clinically significant improvements in the digestive symptoms of people with IBS after twelve weeks.[27]

A second study then found through IgG testing that milk, eggs, wheat, beef, pork and lamb were the most common problem foods in a group of IBS sufferers. After eliminating these and other specific foods there were significant improvements in pain, bloating, bowel habits and general wellbeing after three months and the benefits were still present three months later.[28]

Similar benefits were seen in a year-long study of people who had failed to improve with medical care. After removal of problem foods there were reductions in pain and diarrhoea as well as increased quality of life.[29] And at an examination one year after their last visit most people were still following their specific diet and reporting benefits, although they were also given a probiotic supplement, which may have influenced the results.

The largest and most recent study testing IgG levels in diarrhoea-predominant IBS (IBS-D) sufferers found that IgG levels to certain foods were generally much higher than in people with no symptoms. Of the original 77 people tested, 35 had food intolerances and subsequently eliminated the offending foods. Sure enough, when they were examined again four weeks later their abdominal pain, bloating, diarrhoea, distention, stool shape, general feelings of distress and overall symptoms had improved and remained better when they were examined again six weeks later.[30]

These studies show that, for some people, food intolerances may be an important reason for IBS symptoms. Identifying exactly which foods are problematic can be tricky and time consuming but, ultimately, very beneficial if food intolerance is aggravating your digestive problems.

FOOD ADDITIVES

As the famous food writer Michael Pollan says, 'you don't want to let corporations cook your food for you'. One of the reasons for this is that they use chemicals that you would never use at home. Do you keep aspartame, maltodextrin, monosodium glutamate and polysorbate-80 in your kitchen? I didn't think so, but they are very common in processed foods. And you could even extend this quote to include 'you don't want to let corporations grow your food for you' because that can affect the nutritional quality of your food, too. Would you spray your vegetable patch with toxic chemicals before serving the vegetables to your friends for lunch? No, you would not do that either, but non-organic farming does.

Very recent scientific discoveries have started to uncover potential dangers of common food additives and contaminants that were once thought to be harmless. Because they are in such small quantities in food, pesticides and industrial additives such as sweeteners, flavour enhancers, preservatives and emulsifiers have often been thought to be non-toxic, but new research is changing the way we think about these substances. And at the cutting edge of these discoveries is your digestive system because these new-to-nature chemicals appear to have important adverse effects on your gut bacteria and gastrointestinal health.

Research suggests that food additives can adversely affect gut bacteria and subsequently the integrity of your gastrointestinal barrier, which in turn could cause inflammation and problems with your immune system leading to autoimmune disease. Much of the research in this area is limited to experimental studies, but the results from these investigations are pointing to important implications for human health.[31]

One of the world's leading science journals, *Nature*, published some of the first discoveries in this area, with a study showing that the artificial sweetener aspartame caused changes in the composition and function of gut bacteria in mice, and that these changes were similar to those linked to obesity and diabetes in humans.[32] Similar research has also implicated another common sweetener, sucralose.[33] And the problem does not stop at artificial sweeteners, with many other food additives emerging as a problem. Even food contamination with chemicals from plastic food packaging and agricultural chemicals such as pesticides, which is more common than you might think, could have similar effects.[34]

Most alarmingly, some additives have been linked to changes in gut bacteria that could cause inflammation and the development of gastrointestinal disease. Dietary emulsifiers (carboxymethylcellulose and polysorbate-80) and the sugar maltodextrin, which are very widely used in processed foods, have been shown to destroy the harmonious balance between gut bacteria and the immune system, causing damage to the gut wall and increasing the risk of disease. This occurs even in the very small amounts that we would be exposed to in food, and there is some evidence from studies of people with inflammatory bowel disease suggesting this could be a real concern.[35,36]

Finally, people with chronic fatigue, muscle weakness and pain, headaches and the diverse digestive symptoms of IBS may benefit from avoiding dietary excitotoxins. 'Excitotoxins' is a term given to dietary substances that are toxic to your nervous system. Two of the main excitotoxins are glutamate and aspartate, which are found in the flavouring monosodium glutamate (MSG) and artificial sweetener aspartame, respectively. A clinical study of a group of people with severe muscle pain, fatigue and IBS set out to see if eliminating these from their diet would help. Of those who completed the elimination diet, 84 per cent reported that over 30 per cent of their symptoms improved and when they were challenged with MSG unknowingly they had a significant return of their symptoms.[37]

Taken together, this emerging science suggests the industrial chemicals that are intentionally added to processed food, or might be there due to contamination from plastic packaging or the use of pesticides, could be a very important reason why we see a correlation between increased risk of various diseases as our diet becomes more processed, and that this could be down to the way these industrial chemicals are changing our gut bacteria. While we wait for more research it makes sense to reduce your exposure as much as possible by avoiding processed food, plastic packaging and non-organic food.

HISTAMINE INTOLERANCE

Dietary histamine intolerance has been an important consideration in central Europe for decades but remains relatively unknown elsewhere. A few recent studies have reignited interest in other parts of the world because of the potential benefits of a low-histamine diet.

Histamine intolerance (HIT) is a condition that is characterized by the development of a diverse set of problematic symptoms after the ingestion of histamine-containing foods.[38] Importantly, HIT is thought to be due not solely to dietary histamine exposure, but exposure coupled with insufficient or impaired histamine detoxification, which simply means your body may not be breaking down or 'detoxifying' dietary histamine very well.[39]

Elevations in histamine due to an imbalance between poor detoxification and high dietary exposure can cause allergic type symptoms such as flushing, headaches or skin rash, and gastrointestinal symptoms including diarrhoea and abdominal pain. Actually your body can also make histamine, which is known to cause allergic symptoms, so this should be no surprise from a medical perspective.[40]

Symptoms of histamine intolerance[41]

System	Symptoms
Skin	Flushing Urticaria (skin rash) Itch
Gastrointestinal tract	Nausea/vomiting Abdominal pain Cramps Diarrhoea
Central nervous system	Headache Migraine Dizziness

System	Symptoms
Cardiovascular	Hypotension Tachycardia Cardiac arrhythmi
Respiratory system	Asthma-like symptoms Nasal obstruction Rhinorrhea (runny nose) Rhinitis (hay fever)

Dietary histamine is found at particularly high concentration in aged foods (e.g. cheeses, alcoholic beverages, cured meats, fermented or spoiled foods) where it is produced by bacterial or yeast fermentation of the amino acid histidine to histamine. Other foods, such as citrus, may have the capacity to enhance histamine release even though they contain low levels of histamine themselves.[42]

High-histamine or histamine-provoking foods include the following:

- alcoholic beverages
- oily fish: either processed (tuna, sardine, mackerel) or semi-processed (anchovy, herring)
- shellfish
- cured meats
- pork
- aged cheeses e.g. manchego, parmigiano, cheddar
- fermented foods e.g. tempeh, miso, sauerkraut
- chocolate, vanilla
- fruits: citrus, kiwifruit, nuts and dried fruit, strawberry, pineapple, papaya
- vegetables: spinach, tomato (fresh or sauce), eggplant (aubergine)
- eggs.[43]

Detoxification of dietary histamine normally occurs in intestinal epithelial cells via the enzyme diamine oxidase (DAO) as well as histamine-N-methyl-transferase (HNMT) in the liver. If DAO fails to inactivate histamine it can be absorbed through the gut wall and enter the bloodstream and circulation, where it can cause the typical symptoms of HIT.[44] There have been associations between genetic variations that affect DAO and/or HNMT activity and inflammatory bowel disease, asthma, allergic rhinitis and migraine headache, suggesting increased susceptibility to histamine intolerance in some individuals.[45-48] However, HIT appears to be transient and may depend more on other factors than genetic susceptibility, which tends to have a more modest influence.

The diagnosis of HIT typically requires the presence of two or more symptoms, improvement with a low-histamine diet and/or antihistamines, and the exclusion of food allergies or intolerance. Testing remains controversial as blood and urine histamine is often normal and the usefulness of determining DAO levels or DAO and HNMT genetic variations is unclear.[49]

It is also unclear just how common HIT is, but it appears to be relatively rare.[50] And the only known treatment is a diet low in high-histamine or histamine-provoking foods. Although dietary approaches for HIT have been used clinically for some time, there is not a great deal of evidence scientifically.[51-54] However, a few recent studies found important benefits.

A study in children with chronic abdominal pain found a suspected prevalence of HIT of up to 4 per cent. Children who responded to the histamine-free diet had a significant reduction in their pain symptoms.[55] And another study of children diagnosed with HIT and predominant digestive complaints also reported important clinical benefits from a low-histamine diet.

Major symptoms were widespread abdominal pain, diarrhoea, headache and chronic intermittent vomiting. Less commonly, some patients had rash, asthma, atopic dermatitis or coeliac disease. They followed a low-histamine diet, which resulted in immediate improvement, and only two patients had a recurrence of symptoms (which was less intense), and if symptoms did recur they were then further treated with antihistamine medications or zinc, a natural antihistamine.[56]

Even hayfever medication has been shown to help relive IBS because of its antihistamine effect. In a remarkable study, a group of scientists from the University of Leuven, Belgium, were able to show that histamine has an impact on the pain receptor TRPV1 and could be responsible for the pain seen in IBS. They then tested an antihistamine medication that blocks the effects of histamine on nerves, to see if it would help people with IBS, and found that after twelve weeks there was significantly less abdominal pain. It appears the role of histamine may be more important than has been previously appreciated.[57]

ARE FOOD INTOLERANCES CAUSING YOUR SYMPTOMS?

Not all foods are a problem for all people, and although for some people food intolerances may not be an issue at all, they are certainly worth considering. To determine if food intolerances are contributing to your digestive issues, try the following protocols:

1. **An elimination and re-challenge diet:** One of the best ways to find out if certain foods are a problem is to try an elimination and re-challenge diet. This simply involves removing potential problem foods

from your diet for about four weeks and then slowly re-introducing them one by one to see if they cause problems. This method is often more accurate than blood tests and has been shown to be very helpful for symptom relief. A simple, easy-to-follow elimination and re-challenge program is outlined in the Five Steps to Great Gut Health (see page 159). For a more comprehensive program, it is best to consult with a nutrition professional.

2. **Test for coeliac disease:** Testing for coeliac disease is essential if you have digestive complaints. The standard way to test involves an initial blood test (for IgA anti-tissue transglutaminase antibodies), which is nearly 100 per cent accurate. The diagnosis is then confirmed by a more involved look into your digestive system (upper endoscopy) and a sample of your gut wall (duodenal biopsy), although these may not be necessary if there are obvious clinical symptoms and a positive blood test. Non-coeliac gluten intolerance can only be identified with an elimination and re-challenge diet, which is part of the Five Steps to Great Gut Health (see page159).[58] So, even if your tests say you don't have gluten sensitivity, you may still benefit from a gluten-free diet.

3. **Test for lactose intolerance:** The most commonly used and reliable test for lactose intolerance is a lactose hydrogen breath test. This involves drinking 50 g of lactose (equivalent to about 1 litre of milk) and measuring the levels of hydrogen in your

breath repeatedly over three hours. The test is not completely accurate, as up to 20 per cent of people who are lactose intolerant may not have an increase in breath hydrogen, in which case an elimination and re-challenge diet, detailed in the Five Steps to Great Gut Health (see page 159) may help in diagnosis.

4. **Test for multiple problem foods:** To see if intolerance to multiple foods might be a problem you can do a blood immunoglobulin G (IgG) food intolerance test. This type of test aims to see if you have raised IgG levels to any commonly consumed foods. Raised IgG levels indicate that a particular food may be a problem and thus causing symptoms. IgG testing looks for a wide range of potential problem foods (sometimes more than 80 in a single test). Although controversial and somewhat expensive, identifying and removing foods based on IgG testing has been shown to be very helpful for some people.

How to deal with problem foods

1. **Follow the Five Steps to Great Gut Health:** The five-step plan on page 160 includes an elimination and re-challenge diet to help you identify whether or not some of the most common problem foods are contributing to your symptoms. An elimination and re-challenge diet is a simple and effective way to improve your symptoms if food sensitivities do turn out to be an issue.

2. **Go gluten-free:** The only treatment for coeliac
    disease or gluten sensitivity is a life-long gluten-
    free diet. When commencing a new gluten-free
    lifestyle it's a good idea to consult with a nutrition
    professional as they can advise you on how to go
    gluten-free and maintain a healthy, balanced diet.
    Non-profit coeliac disease societies are an excellent
    source of information too. Going gluten-free is a big
    commitment at first but over time becomes easier
    and eventually a normal part of life.

3. **Go lactose-free:** People who are lactose intolerant
    can still eat dairy foods that are low in lactose or
    lactose-free. Dairy products such as hard cheese
    and natural yoghurt are generally tolerated due to
    their low lactose content and lactose-free milks or
    milk alternatives are available. Generally, people
    can tolerate up to 6 g of lactose in a single serve
    without developing symptoms but you may need to
    find how much you can tolerate through trial and
    error.

4. **Try a low-histamine diet:** If you have symptoms
    that suggest histamine intolerance or you think
    you are reacting to high-histamine foods, you could
    try a low-histamine diet. A nutritionally trained
    health professional could help confirm whether it
    is indeed a case of HIT, and they can also help with
    your food plan as well as additional therapeutic
    considerations. Limiting exposure to histamine-
    containing or histamine-provoking foods as well
    as alcohol, which inhibits intestinal DOA, is the

best place to start. In addition to dietary therapy, nutritional supplementation with nutritional co-factors for DOA and natural antihistamines has been suggested, in particular zinc, vitamin C and vitamin B6 as well as probiotics.[59-61] Several medications are DOA inhibitors and should be reviewed with a health professional to make sure they are not making things worse. And damage to the gut wall, as occurs in inflammatory bowel disease or coeliac disease, may reduce histamine detoxification and should be considered. HIT is often transient and after dietary histamine removal and subsequent reduction in symptoms many people are able to tolerate histamine-containing foods again and return to a normal diet.

5. **Work with a nutrition professional:** With any dietary elimination, whether it's gluten-containing grains, lactose, dairy foods or any number of other problem foods you identify through IgG testing, you should seek advice from a nutrition professional who can advise you on how to make appropriate dietary changes in the long term. This will make things easier and ensures you do not exclude foods without finding suitable, nutritious alternatives.

8

PUT YOUR BACTERIA ON A LOW-CARBOHYDRATE DIET

Carbohydrate-rich foods such as pasta, pizza, biscuits or cookies, cakes, bread, cereals, soft drink (sodas), fruit juice and sweetened dairy products are such common features of our diets that we take them for granted as normal everyday food items. But these foods are all relatively recent phenomena and can have negative effects on your digestion. In fact, a daily diet based on carbohydrate-rich foods — such as cereal, milk and fruit juice for breakfast, a sandwich for lunch and pasta for dinner — could actually be the worst possible thing you could eat if you have digestive problems.

Before delving into the role carbohydrates play in the development of digestive symptoms, it is important to reflect on the fact that 7000 to 10,000 years ago, which is relatively recent in historical terms, none of the aforementioned foods were eaten by humans at all. Prior to the agricultural revolution we lived predominately on lean meats and wild fruits and vegetables, which are naturally very low in sugars. This diet dominated the vast majority of human history, but the rise of agriculture resulted in cereals, dairy products and selectively farmed high-sugar fruits taking over the dinner table. And while fruits were typically enjoyed seasonally, they are now available all year round. More recently our diets have become loaded with refined sugars in all shapes and sizes. The result is a carbohydrate-rich diet linked to chronic diseases such as diabetes and obesity and, as it turns out, poor digestive health.

Technically speaking, carbohydrates are sugars, starches and fibres found in fruits, vegetables, cereal grains and legumes. Many different types of carbohydrates are also added to processed foods with fructose, a type of refined sugar, being one of the most common. There is evidence to suggest your digestive system is simply not built to handle a modern high-carbohydrate diet. For example, in an experiment where healthy people, not even people with IBS, were asked to drink the equivalent amount of fructose found in a typical daily modern diet in a single sitting, over 50 per cent of them experienced bloating, abdominal pain and loose bowels — all classic symptoms of IBS.[1] So it's entirely plausible that, for some people, a high-carbohydrate diet alone could be causing symptoms.

Back in 1931, a pioneering investigation into a condition referred to at the time as 'intestinal carbohydrate dyspepsia' found that in some people, intolerance to dietary carbohydrate resulted in bloating, pain, discomfort and intermittent diarrhoea. The researchers found, through a series of experiments, that the gut bacteria of people with intolerance to dietary carbohydrate was associated with the unusual fermentation of high-carbohydrate foods and excessive gas production. Most remarkably, they found that they were able to treat intestinal carbohydrate dyspepsia with a low-carbohydrate diet and a digestive enzyme supplement.[2] This remarkable work was unfortunately forgotten and the role of carbohydrate intolerance is only now, several decades on, regaining attention.

FRUCTOSE

One specific type of sugar that appears to be a problem for some people with digestive issues is fructose. Over 30 years ago it was first proposed that increasing dietary intakes of fructose could be contributing to digestive problems including bloating, distention, diarrhoea and abdominal pain.[3] In fact, a few studies around this time found that reducing dietary intake of fructose could very effectively relieve these symptoms.[4,5]

Dietary intake of fructose has increased dramatically in the last few hundred years because of an increased consumption of dietary sugars in general. Today, exposure to fructose is now 50 times what it was only 200 years ago.[6] And because high-fructose corn syrup is becoming more popular than cane sugar as a food additive, fructose intakes are continuing to increase.[7] While soft drinks (sodas) are usually blamed as a major source of dietary fructose, they are only one of a number of sources. Baked goods (e.g. breads, breakfast cereals and sweet pastries), fruits, fruit juices and fruit products are all major sources of naturally occurring and added dietary fructose.[8]

The issue with fructose is in part due to how it is absorbed in the digestive system. After you eat fructose there are two ways you can absorb it: the slow way and the fast way. The slow way is very specific to fructose and occurs across your entire bowel. The fast way requires another sugar — glucose — for absorption and occurs much more efficiently. So without sufficient glucose any 'free fructose' may not be absorbed efficiently, and that is where you can run into problems. If there is excessive free fructose hanging around in your gut it can be fermented by your bacteria to cause gas, distention and pain, or may attract water into your bowels causing diarrhoea, spasms and cramping.

Fructose intolerance is actually very common; so common, it is suggested to be quite normal. About 50 per cent of people are unable to completely absorb a test dose of 25 g of fructose, and this is enough to cause gastrointestinal symptoms and distress in otherwise healthy people, not even people with IBS.[9] While it is generally unlikely you are going to drink 25 g of free fructose in one hit, average dietary intakes do range from 11 to 54 g per day, so intolerance to usual dietary amounts of fructose is a real possibility.[10]

Although fructose intolerance is normal and many people who have fructose intolerance don't have IBS, if you do have IBS, fructose intolerance suddenly becomes very relevant, as reducing dietary fructose could be a way to relieve your symptoms. Someone with a healthy gut might get away with consuming fructose whereas someone with IBS, whose gut is very sensitive to gas and distention, is more likely to experience a major exacerbation of their symptoms if they are fructose intolerant. Indeed, testing for fructose intolerance and then reducing exposure to high-fructose foods has been shown to be a very effective way to improve symptoms for some people.

Reducing your intake of high-fructose foods is the standard way to deal with fructose intolerance. Foods that contain large amounts of pure fructose include sweetened cereal and grain products, meal replacements and sports or energy drinks. Foods sweetened with agave nectar, which is predominantly fructose, are also a problem and include a number of health foods and drinks where agave is added as a 'natural' sweetener, although there is nothing particularly natural about consuming a refined sugar syrup. Fructose is also abundant in apples, pears, fruit-juice concentrates, and beverages sweetened with high-fructose corn syrup.

Foods that contain balanced amounts of glucose and fructose, like a banana or maple syrup, are well tolerated, so fructose does not need to be avoided completely.[11] And sorbitol, a type of indigestible sugar found in high amounts in pears, apples and plums, inhibits the absorption of fructose and may add to fructose intolerance.[12]

In addition to fructose intolerance, a number of other dietary carbohydrates, including lactose and certain fibres, can contribute to digestive symptoms, so there is more to this story than just fructose intolerance, but before we go deeper let's have a look at dietary fibre first.

FIBRE

Early studies exploring the role of dietary carbohydrates in digestive diseases most commonly focused on fibre. Based on observations of increased digestive diseases in traditional cultures making the transition from a natural high-fibre diet to modern, processed low-fibre foods, it was assumed that decreases in fibre, which is known to be important for digestive health, were to blame.[13]

However, subsequent tests of high-fibre diets and fibre supplements in people with IBS quickly threw the 'more fibre for healthy bowels' idea into dispute when it was found that increasing fibre has little benefit and in some cases can actually make symptoms a lot worse. A scientific review of many of these studies, seventeen in total, found that in general, fibre supplements were not particularly helpful and could sometimes worsen symptoms.[14]

Interestingly, early investigations exploring the role of food intolerances in IBS discovered that the most problematic foods were often high-fibre cereal grains such as wheat and rye. Onions, which are also very high in indigestible fibre, were also frequently a problem food for IBS sufferers.[15] The elimination of these foods from the diet tended to provide good relief from IBS but at the time it was not understood exactly why.

Shedding light on the fibre conundrum, Professor John Hunter and his group from Cambridge University discovered that the problem might not be down to the fibre itself, but the way it is fermented by gut bacteria. They showed that people with IBS produce a lot more intestinal gas when they eat dietary fibre; they also found that treatment with antibiotics, which kill off your gut bacteria, was able to reduce fermentation and gas production.[16] This remarkable finding suggests that fermentation of fibre by bad gut bacteria, not the fibre itself, could be a major part of the problem.[17]

It has also been found that not just fibre but other types of carbohydrates could be playing a role. About fifteen years ago a research group discovered that placing people with IBS on diets low in the specific sugars lactose, fructose or sorbitol resulted in excellent improvements in symptoms.[18] And a later study found that people on a popular low-carbohydrate weight-loss diet dramatically improved their symptoms within just four weeks.[19] But a specialist group from Monash University in Australia has done the most advanced work in the area of low-carbohydrate diets for IBS — they call their approach the low FODMAP diet.

THE FODMAP APPROACH

Through extensive research a new and very effective dietary approach has been developed for the symptoms of IBS. It is termed the FODMAP diet and is based on the restriction of specific types of poorly digested carbohydrates. This specialized dietary approach restricts foods high in carbohydrates that are poorly absorbed and fermented by gut bacteria (in particular, the sugars fructose and lactose, a class of fibres known as oligosaccharides, and a special group of sugars called polyols). Clinical studies have found that this diet is remarkably effective.[20] In fact, a study comparing the FODMAP approach to the standard dietary advice for IBS issued by the UK National Institute for Health and Care Excellence (NICE) showed that the FODMAP approach was far better for symptom relief including pain, bloating and flatulence.[21]

The FODMAP diet works by restricting carbohydrates that are easily fermented by gut bacteria and subsequently produce gas and distention. The same carbohydrates can also increase the water content of the bowel, further increasing distention and leading to diarrhoea.[22] The pioneers of this approach, Dr Sue Shepherd and Dr Peter Gibson, suggest that modern diets are increasing in FODMAP content due to the overconsumption of refined sugars, diet and low-fat foods, and wheat products, and that this dietary change may be in part responsible for the increases in digestive problems in recent years.[23]

The acronym 'FODMAP' refers to the scientific names for the type of carbohydrates that are restricted on the diet (Fermentable, Oligo-, Di- and Mono-saccharides and Polyols) and was developed so they could be collectively grouped together for the sake of creating a unified name for this concept. From a practical perspective the major carbohydrates that are restricted are free fructose (found in fruits and sweeteners), lactose (from dairy foods), oligosaccharides (from vegetables and cereals) and polyols (in fruits, vegetables and sweeteners). Foods that have the highest levels of these FODMAPs are restricted and substituted with low-FODMAP foods.

Examples of high- and low-FODMAP foods

Food	High	Low
Fruits	Apples, cherries, mango, peaches, pears, plums, prunes, watermelon.	Bananas, berries, grapefruit, grapes, kiwifruit, citrus fruit, passionfruit, papaya (paw paw), rockmelon (cantaloupe).
Vegetables	Artichokes, asparagus, beetroot, Brussels sprouts, broccoli, cabbage, chicory (endive), fennel, garlic, leeks, onions.	Carrot, celery, capsicum (peppers), corn, eggplant (aubergine), green beans, parsnip, pumpkin, tomato.
Cereals	Wheat, rye.	Gluten-free products, spelt.
Legumes	Beans, lentils, chickpeas (garbanzo beans).	
Dairy	Milk, ice cream, soft cheese.	Lactose-free products, hard cheese, butter.
Sweeteners	Fructose, high-fructose corn syrup, honey, sweeteners ending in *ol* (e.g. maltitol, xylitol, sorbitol).	Maple syrup, sugar (sucrose).

While the FODMAP approach has proven to be quite successful, providing good relief to about 75 per cent of people, it is important to note that the approach may not be addressing the underlying cause of IBS. When IBS sufferers are compared to people who are IBS free, there is actually the same amount of fermentation after eating FODMAP-rich foods, which means fermentation itself is quite normal.[24] In fact, fermentation of fibre from fruits, vegetables, legumes and wholegrains is important for digestive health and may help prevent bowel cancer. The difference in IBS is that this normal fermentation process causes distention and pain because the gut is hypersensitive.

So, although the FODMAP approach may be helpful, there are certain drawbacks: it is a restrictive dietary regime that requires supervision and counselling from a trained nutrition professional; the approach also excludes foods that may have important health benefits in the long term and should be seen as a means of symptomatic relief rather than an actual cure. Nevertheless, it can be a very effective way to relieve symptoms, perhaps one of the most effective available.

FAST FOOD FOR BACTERIA

One reason why modern high-carbohydrate diets could lead to digestive problems is that they are providing 'fast food' for your gut bacteria. Small intestinal bacterial overgrowth (SIBO) is very common in IBS and may help explain why high-carbohydrate diets can lead to symptoms. When you eat sugars they are normally fermented by gut bacteria in your large bowel but if you have SIBO, and up to 84 per cent of people with IBS do, sugars can be fermented much earlier on in your small intestine, leading to gas, distention, pain and diarrhoea. Indeed, people who eat a diet high in added sugars and refined carbohydrates and low in fibre tend to have a higher prevalence of SIBO.[25].

Treatment of SIBO with antibiotics has been shown to relieve symptoms, and in one study was also able to improve the digestion and absorption of FODMAPs (lactose, fructose and sorbitol), which in turn reduced fermentation and gas production.[26] So while low-carbohydrate diets such as the FODMAP approach can be beneficial, it is important to keep in mind that an imbalance in your gut bacteria may fundamentally be to blame.

It is also important not to place too much emphasis on one particular dietary approach. As an example, one study comparing the low-FODMAP diet with more traditional advice (a regular meal pattern; avoidance of large meals; and reduced intake of fat, insoluble fibres, caffeine and gas-producing foods such as beans, cabbage, and onions) found that both were just as effective.[27] This is why in the dietary plan in the Five Steps to Great Gut Health we use a combination of both.

THE SPECIFIC CARBOHYDRATE DIET

The Specific Carbohydrate Diet (SCD) has a remarkable evolutionary story. Originally developed for the management of coeliac disease symptoms in the 1950s,[28] the SCD was popularized in the 1980s with the book *Breaking the Vicious Cycle: Intestinal health through diet* for the management of inflammatory bowel disease (IBD). But despite considerable anecdotal reports of benefit, including hundreds of testimonials on Amazon.com, there has not been more rigorous investigation until very recently.[29] The original premise for the diet was very similar to that of the FODMAP diet: the thinking was that restriction of complex carbohydrates and refined sugar from the diet would prevent malabsorption and symptom development. Later the hypothesis was expanded to include the idea that malabsorbed carbohydrates could cause gut bacterial imbalance (dysbiosis) and contribute to the intestinal inflammation of inflammatory bowel disease.

Recently a research group made some striking discoveries concerning the effect of the SCD on the gut bacteria of people with IBD.[30] In the study they examined the effects of the SCD on the gut bacteria and demonstrated for the first time that the diet increased bacterial diversity and increased the abundance of *Faecalibacterium prausnitzii*, an anti-inflammatory and potentially beneficial bacterium. Further, the increase in diversity was maintained long after the diet was finished, suggesting long-term effects of the diet on gut health.

The last few years have seen an increasing number of published scientific reports documenting important clinical benefits of the SCD in IBD patients.[31,32] For example, children with IBD who followed the SCD for an average of fourteen months resolved clinical symptoms and improved or normalized inflammatory markers.[33] And a woman with IBD who was not responding to medication found the SCD diet improved symptoms within three to six months and experienced remission within two years.[34]

In the first proper clinical study of the SCD, nine children with inflammatory bowel disease received dietary treatment over a twelve-week period, then continued the program for up to 52 weeks. Within the first twelve weeks there was a significant improvement with seven of the children (60 per cent) achieving clinical remission by twelve weeks. Sustained clinical remission was seen in six of the seven patients, who remained on the diet to 52 weeks.[35] These reports, while preliminary, are remarkable.

Although the SCD is more frequently used for IBD, there is some indication that it could help with more general digestive symptoms such as bloating and pain, as well as the many other symptoms of IBS. In the only such documented account, a woman with severe IBS symptoms was counselled in a modified version of the SCD by a nutritionist and also prescribed a probiotic as well as being instructed to make her own yoghurt, which she consumed daily. Her symptoms got worse initially, but this is apparently not uncommon, and after around twenty days she eventually experienced an excellent reduction in most of her symptoms that lasted for several months.[36]

Like the low-FODMAP diet, the SCD diet can be very strict and difficult to follow. If you feel it is important to try, it is best to do so under the guidance of a nutritionist or nutritionally trained healthcare professional. Alternatively, there is an easy-to-follow modified version of the SCD in the Five Steps to Great Gut Health on page 192.

How do you know if a high-carbohydrate diet is causing symptoms?

1. **Try a low-carbohydrate diet:** Perhaps the simplest way to find out if too much dietary carbohydrate is a problem is to see if your digestive health improves on a low-carbohydrate diet. Testing for lactose and fructose intolerance first is recommended because if you are not intolerant your diet will be less restrictive. Low-carbohydrate diets have been synonymous with very unhealthy eating in the past but can also be very healthy. A simple and healthy low-carbohydrate eating plan is outlined in the Five Steps to Great Gut Health (page 192).

2. **Test for fructose intolerance:** Fructose intolerance can be tested with a fructose hydrogen breath test, which involves drinking about 35 g of fructose and monitoring the amount of hydrogen gas on your breath repeatedly over the next three hours. High levels of hydrogen indicate fructose intolerance and this can help guide your dietary strategy. If you are fructose intolerant, dietary fructose does not need to be completely eliminated, just reduced to improve your symptoms. An experienced nutrition professional can help you achieve this.

How can you reduce your carbohydrate intake?

1. **Follow the Five Steps to Great Gut Health:** The five-step plan (see page 160) provides you with a healthy eating plan designed specifically to improve your symptoms. The food plan reduces the intake of high-carbohydrate foods that can aggravate digestive issues and will help you identify whether lactose or fructose are a problem. Far from being restrictive, the food plan has plenty of healthy carbohydrate options so you are not left hungry or with no idea what to eat.

2. **Try the low-FODMAP diet:** Another option is to follow the official low-FODMAP diet (see Resources). This diet should, however, be implemented under the supervision of a trained nutrition professional who is familiar with the program and has experience with its implementation. The reason supervision is

important is that the FODMAP approach requires extensive dietary changes that need to be supported with dietary counselling. The approach is also individualized from person to person. So seeing a trained professional is important and will ultimately improve your chances of success.

9

REWIRE THE NERVES OF YOUR GUT–BRAIN AXIS

Stress plays a major role in the development of digestive problems. Stressful events alone can trigger symptoms such as pain and diarrhoea, and if you are chronically stressed symptoms tend to be more severe. About 75 per cent of people with IBS report having serious stress-related symptoms, such as anxiety and depression, and while having digestive issues is itself very stressful, there is good reason to believe that stress can be one of the reasons why you develop symptoms in the first place.[1]

Trauma in early childhood, such as conflict in the family, severe illness, the death of a close family member and mental or physical abuse has been shown to predispose children to the development of IBS later in life.[2] And more recent life stress may play a role as well. In a survey of about 1000 adults without IBS, it was found that people who had anxiety and depression were far more likely to develop IBS in the coming years.[3]

Once you have digestive symptoms, stress is well known to spark flare-ups and make any existing symptoms much worse. Chronic life stresses, especially exposure to situations that cause anxiety, have a potent effect on the severity and intensity of symptoms.[4]

In one study, chronic life stress was found to affect the majority of people with IBS and, in fact, appeared to be the main reason why their symptoms got worse. Researchers assessed people's stress levels and then checked in on them some sixteen months later and found that not one person who was continuously exposed to stress got noticeably better, while only those who said they no longer had any major source of stress in their lives managed to improve.[5] So the effect of stress on digestive symptoms is hugely important, but exactly how does stress affect your digestive system?

THE GUT–BRAIN AXIS

When you face a source of stress your brain reacts by producing hormones that travel throughout your body to help you adapt to the situation. This includes enhancing your mental alertness and increasing oxygen and blood flow to the brain and muscles in what is known as the 'fight-or-flight response'. In our ancient past this response was important for dealing with short-lived threats or challenges to our survival, such as an attack or injury; however, in the modern world the stressors we face are more likely to be daily worries and emotional stress. So, rather than a short-lived stress that allows your reaction to cool off and your body to return to normal, your brain and nervous system are placed under constant pressure, which also means your stress hormones can be travelling around your body at unusually high levels for long periods of time.[6]

If you have ever felt chronic fatigue, worry, anxiety, irritability, sleeplessness or are simply unable to cope, there is a good chance you have suffered from chronic stress, as these are some of the most common symptoms. What you may not be aware of is just how dangerous the effects of chronic stress are. The way we view stress has changed dramatically over the last few decades and it is now clear that chronic stress can lead to an endless array of health problems including anxiety disorders, major depression, insomnia, infections, allergies, autoimmune disease, diabetes, weight gain, heart disease, chronic fatigue syndrome and, of course, digestive problems.[7]

Your physical response to stress is orchestrated by parts of your nervous system known as the hypothalamic-pituitary-adrenal (HPA) axis and the sympathetic nervous system (SNS), which together are the two major stress response systems. The HPA axis is made up of three major parts: the hypothalamus and the pituitary gland, which are found in your brain; and your adrenal glands, which sit on top of your kidneys. Activation of the HPA axis triggers a domino effect release of hormones from the hypothalamus to the pituitary and then all the way down to your adrenal glands which then produce the stress hormone cortisol. The SNS, on the other hand, is made up of nerve fibres that extend from your brain and branch out through your body and is responsible for the fight-or-flight response and release of the stress hormone adrenaline.

Although most people are familiar with the basic fight-or-flight response, the true dynamics of chronic stress are less appreciated. Chronic stress first results in an overactive stress response (or more specifically, a hyperactivity of the HPA axis), which then over time eventually becomes exhausted and under-functioning.[8] When you are in the early stages of overactivity, it's like your nervous system is constantly 'wired' and hyperreactive, while the later stage is quite the opposite and appropriately referred to as adrenal burnout. Physically and mentally, there are symptoms that define this progression: in the early stages of hyperactivity you may be strung out, anxious and unable to sleep, and in the latter stages you may suffer from extreme fatigue, oversleeping and a flat, exhausted type of depression.[9]

A great deal of study into the functioning of the nervous systems of people with IBS has been undertaken and it is becoming clear that people with IBS tend to have a chronic hyperactivity of their nervous systems. When tested, levels of the stress hormones cortisol and adrenaline are often greater in IBS sufferers even when they are relatively stress free, and when exposed to a stressful event the subsequent production of these hormones tends to be much higher.[10,11]

A major source of stress for most people is public speaking and this is often used in stress research to see what effect stress is having on the body. As one study using this method discovered, women with IBS who were told that they had to deliver a public speech the next day tended to produce much more of the stress hormone cortisol than women who were IBS free. They also had much worse sleep patterns, which is similarly related to hyperactivity of your nervous system.[12]

The increased level and production of stress hormones seen in IBS undoubtedly directly influences symptoms. Several experiments have shown that when people with IBS are stressed, they tend to have increased pain sensitivity in the colon.[13] So if your nervous system is in a state of alarm, it appears your digestive system is too, and this is due to the direct influence of stress hormones in the tissues, muscles and nerve fibres that make up your gastrointestinal tract.

Your brain and digestive system are in constant communication via what is referred to as the gut–brain axis.

Your brain, through various hormones and nerve pathways, controls normal digestive function. Stress hormones, such as cortisol and adrenaline, can influence your digestive function via the nerves that travel directly from your brain to your gut. This communication superhighway travels both ways, which means digestive problems can affect your mood and behaviour too.[14] For example, brain imaging studies have consistently shown that people with IBS tend to have a heightened response to gastrointestinal pain in areas of the brain that are responsible for symptoms of stress and emotional arousal.[15]

The most intriguing example of how your digestive health can affect your brain and behaviour comes from studies of gut bacteria. Early experiments found that the introduction of even very low levels of unhealthy bacteria in mice was enough to trigger anxiety-like symptoms.[16] This remarkable discovery suggested that gut bacteria might be directly causing anxiety symptoms via the gut–brain axis. Sure enough, a subsequent study in mice was able to demonstrate that the administration of healthy bifidobacteria reduced anxiety through direct activation of a nerve pathway that runs from your digestive system to your brain.[17]

Human clinical studies have also found that certain probiotic supplements can reduce stress and anxiety. In a report published in the *British Medical Journal* a group of people taking probiotics for 30 days reported lower levels of stress-related symptoms such as depression, anger and anxiety. When tested they also had lower levels of the stress hormone cortisol.[18] The discovery that the balance of bacteria in your digestive system could be affecting your mood is hugely important, as low levels of good bacteria, especially bifidobacteria, and high levels of bad bugs, is a common finding in IBS sufferers.

THE STRESS OF LIVING WITH DIGESTIVE ILLNESS

Living with digestive symptoms can be a traumatic experience. Whereas people might normally experience 'butterflies' in their stomach if they are nervous, people with IBS often experience a thunderstorm of pain, bloating and changes in bowel motions. Because the gut is hypersensitive, even small amounts of stress can be upsetting to the extent that it can literally be crippling, leaving people unable to work or enjoy daily life.

Pain and other symptoms can provoke anxiety, depression and mental exhaustion. Diarrhoea or a sense of urgency, for example, can cause extreme worry because of the possibility of not making it to the bathroom on time. Bloating and distention can be unsightly and embarrassing, and constant pain can have a tremendous impact on mental health and wellbeing.

Coping with symptoms can be very difficult and a fear of symptoms can stop people from engaging in social activities. They end up feeling despair and are depressed because they think the condition is out of control. Family and social relationships are frequently affected, as can be marriages and sexual relationships. People can be afraid to eat at work for fear of symptoms and may withdraw socially, causing further anxiety, anger, guilt and shame.

Your mind, gut, emotions and experiences all interconnect to create important intertwined relationships that need to be considered if you are going to improve your symptoms. This understanding of how emotions influence digestive symptoms and how digestive symptoms can conversely influence emotions via the gut–brain axis is central to how mind–body therapies can improve your physical and emotional health.

How do you know if stress is linked to your symptoms?

1. **Keep a diary:** A daily diary is a simple way to identify a relationship between stressful events and subsequent symptoms. The Five Steps to Great Gut Health includes a symptom diary and instructions on how to identify whether stress is exacerbating your digestive problems (see Your Daily Symptom Diary on page 183). After recording your digestive symptoms and any stressful events at the end of each week you can see if there is a relationship between the score in your symptom diary and these questions.

2. **See a health professional:** Often people have symptoms of anxiety or depression that are significant enough to require additional care and treatment. If you have had long-term feelings of sadness and hopelessness, have lost interest in the things you used to enjoy, feel 'tearful', restless, constantly 'on edge', have difficulty concentrating or are regularly irritable, and these symptoms are significantly affecting your daily life, you should consider seeking medical advice. It is also a good idea to seek the advice of a health professional who practises natural medicine, so you can try natural solutions that may improve your symptoms.

What can you do to reduce the stress of IBS?

1. **Follow the Five Steps to Great Gut Health:** The five-step plan (page 160) details some practical steps you can take to help manage stress more effectively and improve your gastrointestinal and emotional symptoms. Because your symptoms are inextricably linked to your mental and emotional health, basic stress-management strategies are important for your recovery.

2. **Try cognitive behavioural therapy:** Cognitive behavioural therapy (CBT) is the best-studied mind–body therapy for IBS and has been shown to be effective for improving gastrointestinal symptoms, psychological distress and overall quality of life.[19,20] CBT works by progressively changing behaviours that perpetuate symptoms while instilling new adaptive behaviours, such as relaxation or meditation, to effectively manage the illness. Typically, a trained therapist facilitates CBT over ten to twelve sessions, or alternatively, the self-help CBT workbook *Controlling IBS the Drug-free Way: A 10-step plan for symptom relief* by Dr Jeffrey Lackner has been shown to be just as effective.[21]

3. **Try hypnotherapy:** Specially developed gut-focused hypnotherapy has been shown in a number of studies to improve gastrointestinal symptoms by about 50 per cent by reducing psychological symptoms and improving general life functioning.[22] Most people seem to respond well and benefits

appear to be maintained for some years afterwards. The treatment involves a practitioner inducing you into a hypnotic state of deep relaxation and then guiding you through therapeutic suggestions, including muscle relaxation, further relaxation of your gastrointestinal system and strengthening your inner resilience, through visualization.

4. **Try other mind–body therapies:** A number of mind–body therapies have been investigated including psychodynamic psychotherapy, biofeedback therapy, progressive muscle relaxation, yoga, meditation, mindfulness, relaxation and stress management. All these have shown some indication of benefit, in particular psychodynamic psychotherapy. If a particular mind–body therapy appeals to you it is worth seeing if regular practice or treatment helps.

10

RESET YOUR DIGESTIVE CLOCK

Poor quality sleep is one of the most common and troubling problems affecting people with digestive symptoms and has a huge effect on wellbeing and quality of life.[1] Studies have consistently shown that an alarmingly large number of people with digestive symptoms and pain suffer so badly that it interferes with their sleep. But to say that poor sleep is merely a consequence of digestive problems would be ignoring evidence that suggests a bad night's sleep can actually be a cause of bad bowels.[2]

A number of scientists now think that, for some people at least, sleep problems could actually be a cause of their digestive issues and over the last twenty years some important discoveries have been made to suggest this may well be the case. Although it is still not entirely clear whether sleep disturbances could cause IBS, or if IBS causes sleep disturbances (most likely it's a combination of both), it is clear that getting a good night's sleep could make a tremendous difference to your symptoms.

One of the first studies to suggest that poor sleep could

be linked to IBS used a dietary record to see if there was a correlation between how well people were sleeping the night before and the severity of IBS symptoms the following day. This simple investigation revealed for the first time that people who reported particularly bad sleep were much more likely to have worse symptoms the following day. And, tellingly, the same study also revealed that if people had a good night's sleep, their symptoms were subsequently much better.[3]

Since this report, poor sleep has been strongly associated with IBS symptoms in a number of investigations. For example, in a large survey of people it was discovered that those who reported having difficulty sleeping as little as four times a month were much more likely to have digestive complaints including upper abdominal pain and discomfort, nausea, reflux symptoms, diarrhoea, loose stools or constipation.[4] Similarly, a study with a group of nurses found that those on disruptive rotating shift work were much more likely to have abdominal pain than those who had more stable working hours and sleeping patterns.[5]

Studies involving sleep restriction and the subsequent assessment of gastrointestinal changes have also been revealing. A study into a group of healthy IBS-free adults found that sleep deprivation for 40 hours increased sensitivity to pain in the same way that IBS sufferers have heightened pain sensitivity. This important finding suggests that lack of sleep may be causing or exacerbating pain. It was also discovered in this same study that 'recovery sleep' was able to reduce sensitivity to pain.[6] While the sleep deprivation in this experiment was extreme, heightened pain sensitivity has also been reported in people who had their sleep reduced to four hours for just one night, which is closer to what someone with insomnia might get, so a bad night's sleep may well lead to increased gastrointestinal pain, characteristic of IBS.[7]

There is also evidence to show that IBS sufferers may have low levels of a hormone that is important for enabling a good night's sleep — melatonin. The natural production of melatonin is triggered in your brain in response to the darkness of night and is known to play an important role in aiding sleep. When taken as a dietary supplement, melatonin is known to help people fall asleep faster and to get a better, more satisfying night's rest.[8]

Interestingly, melatonin has many other functions in the body beyond its role in sleep, including in the gastrointestinal tract. In fact, melatonin is not only produced in your brain, your gastrointestinal system is also an important place where melatonin is produced in your body. Melatonin's role in the gastrointestinal system is poorly understood but it appears to play a role in normal muscle contractions and reducing pain and inflammation.[9]

People with abdominal pain and IBS have been shown to have lower levels of melatonin compared to people without any symptoms, as well as evidence of a disruption in their natural circadian rhythm.[10] Melatonin is available in some countries as a safe, relatively inexpensive dietary supplement and it has been studied in people with IBS who also have sleep problems, with very promising results. In one such study, after two weeks of taking 3 mg of melatonin, IBS sufferers had a significant reduction in abdominal pain, reductions in pain sensitivity and improvements in gastrointestinal function.[11] And in two more studies, people taking 3 mg of melatonin over an eight-week period had significant improvements in their IBS symptoms compared to placebo. They also reported improvements in their sleep as well as reductions in the symptoms of anxiety and depression and improvements in overall quality of life.[12,13]

So melatonin seems to work very well for reducing digestive

symptoms, but why would your natural production of melatonin be low in the first place? Well, the main reason is related to your age-old connection to the Earth's natural day and night cycles. From an evolutionary perspective, we have always been exposed to natural day and night cycles which have had a strong influence on how our body functions. Many metabolic processes, including the activity of organs such as the digestive system and the production of hormones (such as melatonin), respond to natural dark and light cycles. Our 'biological clock', however, has been disrupted with the recent (in evolutionary terms) use of electric lighting at night and lack of natural sunlight during the day as a consequence of spending unusual amounts of time indoors under dim artificial lights.

The way your biological clock works is fairly straightforward. When your eyes (or more specifically the part of your eye called the retina) are exposed to complete darkness, your pineal gland (located in your brain) produces melatonin. Melatonin could be viewed as the 'arm of your biological clock' as it regulates your body's day and night cycles and tells your body what time it is.[14] Conversely, when your eyes are exposed to light, melatonin production is suppressed.[15] Even very small changes in evening light exposure can reduce melatonin concentrations, so electric lighting, television viewing, and the use of digital devices late into the evening appears to be the most likely reason why your melatonin might be low, aside from shift work or disruption due to long plane flights across time zones.[16]

When your biological clock is out of time your nervous system may also be affected, which helps explain why melatonin supplements not only relieve IBS symptoms and insomnia, but anxiety and depression as well. It may be that by restoring your natural production of melatonin you will, in turn, calm down your nervous system. A chronic overactivity of your nervous system has been strongly linked to difficulty sleeping and insomnia, and people with IBS have been found to have higher levels of rapid eye movement (REM) sleep, which indicates a high level of nervous system arousal during the night.[17,18] It has been proposed that one of the ways melatonin works is by reducing the activity of your nervous system, with some evidence to show that melatonin can improve nervous system function and reduce symptoms of chronic stress, in addition to improving sleep and IBS symptoms.[19]

So a bad night's sleep can cause bad bowels and vice versa. Making sure you are getting a good night's sleep could make a big difference to your gastrointestinal symptoms as well as your mood, emotions and overall wellbeing.

How do you know if lack of sleep is causing your symptoms?

1. **Do you have insomnia?** You should be getting about seven to eight hours of sleep each night, as this is considered ideal for adults (children need longer, and in older age it's a little less). However, many people don't get this much sleep and suffer from insomnia, which is not simply a lack of sleep. If you have: a) difficulty falling asleep; b) difficulty remaining asleep; c) wake up too early in the morning; or d) wake up feeling unrefreshed and tired, there is a good chance you have insomnia and that this is contributing to your symptoms.

2. **Test your melatonin levels:** It is possible to see if your melatonin production is low by performing

a simple test that involves taking a sample of your saliva. This is a non-invasive and accurate way to assess whether or not you have a disrupted biological clock and low melatonin production. It is best to speak to a healthcare professional about the suitability of this test. Alternatively, you could try resetting your biological clock or taking melatonin and see if your symptoms improve (see below).

What can you do to improve your sleep?

1. **Reset your body clock:** When you are exposed to complete darkness your pineal gland produces melatonin and conversely, when your eyes are exposed to light, melatonin production is suppressed. Exposing your eyes to bright light in the morning, and limiting your exposure to artificial light late at night can reset your biological clock and restore natural melatonin production. To reset your rhythm: a) spend more time in the dark, extending the dark period at night to nine or ten hours if possible; b) black out your bedroom with some good blinds or blackout curtains; c) reduce your screen viewing time in the evening (including devices such as televisions, mobile phones, tablets, e-readers and laptops); d) practise quiet wakefulness (if you do wake during the night, do not turn on the lights as this will turn off your melatonin production); and e) catch the sunrise (exposing your eyes to bright early morning light helps restore melatonin levels; if the sun is not available, try a dawn-simulating light).

2. **Try melatonin:** Melatonin is a safe and relatively inexpensive dietary supplement. Unfortunately, in some countries (including Australia and the United Kingdom) melatonin is only available on prescription, in which case you will need to speak to a licensed healthcare professional about its suitability. Studies have generally found that 3 mg of melatonin taken at bedtime over about eight weeks can be beneficial. If you are going to purchase melatonin on the internet or abroad, make sure it's from a reputable company and it is the synthetic form of the actual hormone (not the homeopathic type).

3. **Try music therapy:** The sound of relaxing music distracts your mind, induces a physical state of calmness, lowers stress hormones and has been shown to be effective for insomnia. Most studies have found increasing benefit from listening to relaxing music for 45 minutes before bed daily, after a period of three weeks. A wide variety of relaxing music has been found to be effective, such as slow jazz, piano, classical and electronic music, with or without lyrics. Find slow, peaceful, calm music you enjoy then follow these steps: a) lie in bed at your usual bedtime with a comfortable room temperature, wearing comfortable nightclothes, with the lights out and your eyes closed; b) play the music at a comfortable volume; c) use earphones if preferred; and d) do not worry about turning off the music to fall asleep, just let it play.

11

GET ON A DIGESTIVE FITNESS PROGRAM

Regular exercise is vital to your health. In fact, your body does not function properly without it and, although it may not be obvious, this includes your digestive system. Many people, however, do not exercise regularly and this can have an important effect on digestive function, leading to problems such as bloating and constipation.

Physical activity has a profound effect on your physiology, influencing hundreds of cellular processes in multiple organ systems throughout your entire body.[1] This widespread effect of physical activity is why it can prevent and even effectively treat so many health problems — obesity, heart disease, type 2 diabetes and various cancers, to name a few.

And the health of your digestive system is influenced by how much exercise you are getting as well, with evidence linking low physical activity to colon cancer, constipation, bloating, reflux, peptic ulcers, gall stones, diverticular disease (the formation of pouches within the bowel wall) and IBS.[2] Importantly, regular exercise can also reduce many common complaints associated with IBS, such as depression, anxiety, chronic fatigue and fibromyalgia.

The problem is that although you are physically designed to be active, our modern technology and lifestyle has resulted in exercise changing from a necessity of daily living to something that is entirely optional. Your ancestors evolved in an environment where physical activity was essential for survival; they depended on hunting and gathering for the acquisition of food and probably exercised at a level four to five times that of the average person today.[3] In stark contrast, we modern humans hardly exercise at all. In fact, at least 60 per cent of the global population fails to achieve the minimum recommendation of 30 minutes of moderate-intensity physical activity, such as brisk walking, daily.[4]

Along with stress management and healthy eating, regular exercise has long been recommended for people with digestive complaints but only recently has lack of exercise been seriously considered as a possible cause of IBS. This may be due to the assumption that IBS sufferers are simply less active because of the restrictions IBS can place on day-to-day life. Fear of diarrhoea, or bloating and pain can make it tough to engage in even simple activities like going for a walk. Indeed, IBS sufferers are often less physically active but in some cases this may in part explain the development of digestive problems in the first place.

One of the first indications that increasing physical activity may help resolve digestive illness came from a study that assessed the therapeutic effects of an educational class focusing on diet, stress management and exercise. When analyzing the effects of the lifestyle changes people made after the class, it was found that increases in exercise corresponded with significant reduction in abdominal pain when symptoms were reviewed six months later.[5]

Following on from this promising discovery, a subsequent study was undertaken to see if daily physical activity levels corresponded with IBS symptoms, with the aim to shed more light on the relationship between exercise and digestive symptoms. Over the course of the study a group of women completed IBS symptom and physical activity diaries, which were then analyzed to see if there were any important relationships. Firstly, the study results revealed that IBS sufferers were generally much less active than women who were IBS free. More striking though, was the finding that women who were more active were less likely to have specific symptoms, such as the feeling of incomplete evacuation following a bowel movement, and they also had lower levels of fatigue.[6]

The idea that low levels of physical activity may contribute to digestive symptoms has been further supported by studies that specifically looked at the effects of exercise in IBS sufferers. These investigations have revealed that increasing activity with light exercise, such as walking for 20 to 60 minutes, four to five times a week, decreases IBS symptoms significantly within three months. More specifically, regular exercise has been shown to decrease overall IBS symptoms, especially constipation, and improve quality of life.[7,8]

The effects of increasing your physical activity levels do, however, appear to be modest and may be more effective if you have predominant bloating and constipation. Regular exercise has been shown to be very effective at relieving abdominal bloating; when you are inactive you tend to retain more gas in your digestive system and if you are prone to bloating and distention this can make things uncomfortable. Increasing your activity levels can increase the normal clearance of gas from your gut, reducing distention and improving your symptoms.[9]

In the same way physical activity improves the clearance of gas and reduces bloating and distention, it also improves regularity and relieves constipation. Regular physical activity is very important for maintaining healthy elimination. In a study of adults with chronic constipation it was found that a daily exercise program consisting of 30 minutes of brisk walking and about 10 minutes of home-based flexibility and strength exercises was able to significantly improve constipation, reducing troublesome symptoms such as hard stools, a feeling of incomplete defecation and straining. Using X-ray imaging, the researchers found that the exercise program was able to significantly improve colon transit time, which helps explain these benefits.[10]

So regular physical activity is essential not only for good health, but healthy digestive function. Studies show that increasing your physical activity can result in reductions in pain, bloating, distention, constipation, hard stools, incomplete bowel movements and straining. In addition, regular physical activity can boost your mood, relieve depression and anxiety and increase your energy levels, making it an important way to improve your IBS symptoms and general wellbeing.

Is physical inactivity contributing to your symptoms?

For most people, regular physical activity is going to be an important step towards optimal digestive health. Although it may not be the main cause, and the effects of exercise alone may not solve your digestive issues, being active is an important part of maintaining a healthy lifestyle.

1.   **Are you active?** Most health guidelines suggest that you should be achieving a level of physical activity equivalent to 30 minutes of brisk walking most days of the week, and more than this is only beneficial. If you are not achieving this, and most people are not, it's possible that your gastrointestinal symptoms will improve with an increase in daily activity levels.

2.   **Check your steps:** Using a pedometer (a small electronic device that measures your steps) or fitness tracker it is possible to work out where you sit on the physical activity scale. Carry the pedometer around for three days and record the number of steps you take each day then compare them to these figures to work out how active you are:

     •   sedentary = fewer than 5000 steps
     •   low activity = 5000–7499 steps
     •   moderately active = 7500–9999 steps
     •   active = 10,000–12,500 steps
     •   highly active = 12,500 steps or more.

How can you increase your daily physical activity?

1.   **Get moving:** Exercise shouldn't be a chore; make it fun, find an activity you enjoy (e.g. swimming, tennis, yoga, squash, cycling, aerobics, self-defence) and stick with it. Consider recruiting someone to join you so you can keep each other motivated. Walking is a great place to start because it's enjoyable, easy and requires minimal effort. If you haven't exercised for quite a while take it

slowly and stay motivated, as it will become easier in time. Walking requires no initial cost although comfortable walking shoes are recommended to support your feet and protect your knees and back.

2. **The 10,000-step challenge:** The 10,000-step challenge is an effective way to help you find ways to build regular physical activity into your daily life. First, using a pedometer or fitness tracker identify your daily step number then find ways to increase your activity levels to reach a daily target of 10,000 steps. These may include parking further away from where you are going and walking the rest of the way, walking to the corner store each morning for the paper, taking a 10- to 15-minute walk on your lunch break or walking regularly with friends, family, a dog or a local walking club. Keeping a daily diary of your steps is a great way to track your achievements. After a few months you will find that the extra activity simply becomes a normal part of your everyday life and you can ditch the pedometer.

3. **Try yoga:** Yoga has been shown to reduce gastrointestinal symptoms in IBS sufferers within about four weeks of practice and has the added benefit of being an excellent way to reduce stress. Consider joining a yoga class — there will likely be a centre near where you live. If a yoga class is inaccessible, instructional videos can be a very effective way to learn, as studies have shown they can still improve IBS.[11,12]

PART 3

THE FIVE STEPS TO GREAT GUT HEALTH

11

THE FIVE-STEP PLAN FOR
DIGESTIVE HEALTH

The Five Steps to Great Gut Health is a simple, structured
approach to getting your digestive symptoms under control
quickly. The previous chapters are necessary reading, as they
will help you identify more personalized treatments specifically
relevant to you. However, the following plan has simple and
broad-sweeping aims that will likely benefit most people —
natural symptom relief, improving gut bacteria, helping to
improve nervous system health, a specially formulated food plan
and advice on staying symptom free.

Start the five-step plan in order. First you will need to review
which natural supplements you think might work best for
you and start using them (Step 1). Then you will need to start
using probiotics, prebiotics and/or foods that improve your gut
bacteria (Step 2). Once you have started on these steps you can
move on to incorporating the advice on mind–body therapies for
stress management and making dietary changes (Steps 3 and 4).
These later steps are a lot more involved and will require some
forethought and preparation. Finally, once you have finished
these initial recommendations and started to improve your

symptoms, which can happen fast but will typically take about three months, you can start considering how you are going to remain symptom free (Step 5).

You may experience some mild increases in symptoms with some of the initial steps over the first few days, but these typically subside as your digestive system finds its balance again. There is a good chance you will experience a significant reduction in your symptoms with just the initial prescriptions alone. Relief may occur instantly, but it is important to allow about four weeks.

The mind–body therapies will help you to calm down your nervous and digestive systems, while the dietary changes will quickly reduce exposure to any foods that could be contributing to your problem and then help you identify and eliminate them for good. These later lifestyle and dietary changes will help you reduce symptoms in the long term, so hopefully you will no longer rely on taking the natural supplements as often.

Although a little commitment is required, the benefits should be quite quick and you will learn lifestyle and dietary changes that ensure the effects are long lasting.

STEP 1: GET FAST SYMPTOM RELIEF

Pain, diarrhoea, constipation, bloating, distention and cramping are terrible symptoms to have to deal with daily. The first step in the Five Steps to Great Gut Health program is to start reducing symptoms as quickly as possible because any relief you get is going to make following the rest of the plan a lot easier and life in general a lot more manageable.

A number of natural medicines have been shown to be effective for IBS symptoms, in particular peppermint oil, digestive enzymes, artichoke leaf extract, herbal medicines and aloe vera juice. Not all of these will work for everyone and, in most cases, they will not completely resolve your symptoms, but they can reduce them significantly and make life a lot better. Below is a quick reference guide to natural medicines to help you choose which ones might suit you best. More detailed descriptions and dosage instructions follow below.

Quick guide to natural medicines for symptom relief

	Why use this in particular?	How much should I take?	How long does it take to work?
Peppermint oil	Especially effective for flatulence, abdominal pain and distention.	1–2 enteric-coated capsules three times daily.	Immediately and up to 8 weeks for significant pain relief.
Digestive enzymes	If symptoms are worse after eating, such as cramping, bloating, urgency, diarrhoea and pain.	1–3 tablets or capsules *per trigger meal.*	Immediately after trigger meals up to 6 weeks.
Artichoke leaf extract	Particularly effective for cramping and abdominal pain.	1–2 capsules or tablets with meals daily.	After 2–3 weeks and up to 6–8 weeks.
Herbal medicine mixtures	Reduces overall symptoms including abdominal pain.	Follow instructions.	Up to 2–4 weeks.
Aloe vera inner-leaf juice	Improves regularity and reduces discomfort.	100 ml twice daily.	Up to 4 weeks.

Peppermint oil

The use of peppermint as a natural digestive aid dates back to ancient Greece. Minthe was the name of a beautiful nymph who, in Greek mythology, was transformed into a plant by Pluto's jealous wife after she caught her husband's affections. Pluto could not reverse the spell so instead gave her a sweet smell that would permeate the garden. Peppermint oil is obtained by steam distillation of the fresh peppermint plant.

How it works: Peppermint oil has been shown to relax the muscles in the gastrointestinal tract, which explains its ability to reduce muscle spasms, cramping and pain.[1,2] In fact, peppermint oil appears to be just as effective as muscle-relaxant drugs for people with IBS.[3] Experimental studies have shown that peppermint oil could also act as a natural antibiotic against a range of bacteria including *Helicobacter pylori*, *Staphylococcus aureus* and *Escherichia coli*, so it may be that peppermint oil helps balance your gut bacteria by killing off bad bugs too.[4]

Clinical effects: More than ten clinical studies have investigated the effects of peppermint oil in people with IBS, with significant beneficial effects demonstrated across these studies. Peppermint oil has been shown to improve a wide range of symptoms including diarrhoea, bloating and constipation, but it is particularly effective for abdominal pain and discomfort.[5]

Safety: Peppermint oil is extremely well tolerated at the recommended dosage and is very unlikely to cause side effects. Perianal burning and nausea are rarely reported and the safety of peppermint oil during pregnancy is not known, so it is best to avoid if you are pregnant. Peppermint oil may interact with some medications, so if you are taking prescription medications check with your doctor before use.[6]

Recommended dose: Generally, studies have shown that 1–2 enteric-coated capsules (0.2–0.4 ml) three times daily will produce beneficial effects. Often benefits are noticed within the first few days but the best results, particularly for pain relief, have been noticed after about eight weeks of continued use.

Digestive enzymes

Each day, a normally functioning pancreas produces up to 2 litres of pancreatic juice, a concentrated source of enzymes that break down your food, especially fats. If your enzyme production is too low you can end up with nutrient deficiencies, malabsorption, pain and diarrhoea and, for this reason, digestive enzyme supplements have been used for several decades to treat a number of serious digestive diseases. Only recently have digestive enzyme supplements been shown to reduce symptoms, such as cramping, bloating, diarrhoea and abdominal pain.

How they work: When taken with a meal, digestive enzyme supplements increase the concentration of enzymes in your gut so you can break down your food more effectively. The enzyme lipase breaks down fat, amylase breaks down carbohydrate and protease breaks down protein. Taken with a high-fat meal they have been shown to reduce bloating, gas and a feeling of fullness.[7] Digestive enzymes improve IBS symptoms in people who are not digesting fats well and it is possible that they also work by breaking down foods that usually trigger symptoms so they are no longer a problem, such as onions or spicy foods.

Clinical effects: Digestive enzymes work best for symptoms that are aggravated by eating, especially foods that commonly trigger symptoms such as meals away from home, spicy foods, dairy products, cabbage, fried food, peppers, tomatoes and onions. Clinical studies have shown that when taken with food, especially trigger foods, digestive enzymes can reduce cramping, bloating, urgency, stool frequency, diarrhoea and abdominal pain. They seem to work best for diarrhoea-predominant IBS (IBS-D).

Safety: Side effects due to digestive enzyme supplements are rare and supplementation is considered very safe. The most commonly reported side effects are headaches, dizziness, abdominal pain and flatulence but these generally occur in less than 6 per cent of people. Safety in pregnancy is unclear, so digestive supplements are best avoided.[8]

Recommended dose: Studies that have shown benefit have used animal-derived products at a dose of between 8000–24,000 USP (United States Pharmacopeia) units of lipase per meal, or about 1–3 capsules or tablets. If you would prefer to use a vegetarian enzyme, it is best to follow the label recommendations, which is usually about 1–2 capsules or tablets per meal. Unfortunately, there is tremendous variety in available products, so make sure it contains lipase at the recommended dose of lipase units (LU), and has at least the enzymes amylase and protease as well.

Artichoke leaf

Artichoke (*Cynara scolymus*) is a common vegetable native to the Mediterranean, which was cultivated by the ancient Greeks and Romans. Although widely consumed as a vegetable, the leaves are a popular folk remedy for digestive problems, in particular dyspepsia or heartburn. Modern research has confirmed the beneficial effects of artichoke leaves for dyspepsia, and because people who suffer from dyspepsia often also have symptoms such as diarrhoea, constipation, bloating and abdominal pain, it is perhaps not surprising that artichoke leaves have shown promise as a treatment for IBS as well.

How it works: Artichoke leaf has been shown to act as an anti-spasmodic, reducing muscle spasms in the gastrointestinal tract.[9] In addition, the leaves have been shown to stimulate bile production.[10] Bile is secreted into the digestive system by your gall bladder to help digest fats, so it may be that artichoke works in part by aiding digestion.

Clinical effects: In people with IBS, artichoke has been shown to reduce abdominal pain, abdominal cramps, bloating, flatulence, diarrhoea and constipation.[11,12] And in people with more general digestive complaints such as fat intolerance, dyspepsia and chronic constipation, artichoke may significantly reduce nausea, abdominal pain, loss of appetite, constipation and flatulence.[13]

Safety: Less than 1 per cent of people using artichoke may experience mild flatulence or hunger, but these symptoms disappear if you reduce the dose; otherwise there are no known side effects. Because artichoke leaf can improve bile production you should speak to your doctor before using it if you have gall bladder or liver disease. Safety in pregnancy has not been studied, so it is best avoided. There are no known drug interactions but if you are on medication check with your doctor first.

Recommended dose: Clinical studies have found that 640 mg of artichoke leaf extract taken one to three times daily is most effective; this is typically the equivalent of 1–2 capsules taken two to three times daily for most products. Try taking 320 mg twice daily then increase the dose slowly if you need to. The capsules should be taken with water at meal times. Although artichoke might work for you immediately, the best effects have been noticed after six to eight weeks of daily use.

Herbal medicine mixtures

Plants have been used as medicines for thousands of years and are still widely used around the world today. Herbs contain a complex mixture of bioactive compounds making them different from pharmaceutical drugs, which tend to be based on a single chemical with a very specific action. In traditional herbal therapy a number of herbs are often combined to increase the effects of the treatment.[14]

Several recent studies have shown that various herbs from a range of traditional cultures have been shown to be beneficial for digestive health, including candytuft (*Iberis amara*), peppermint (*Mentha piperita*), chamomile (*Anthemis nobilis*), licorice (*Glycyrrhiza glabra*), angelica (*Angelica archangelica*), caraway (*Carum carvi*), milk thistle (*Silybum marianum*), lemon balm (*Melissa officinalis*), greater celandine (*Chelidonium majus*), peony (*Paeonia lactiflora*), cinnamon (*Cinnamomum zeylanicum*), jujube berries (*Ziziphus jujuba*), ginger (*Zingiber officinale*), atractylodes (a Chinese herb), orange peel and ledebouriella root (*Ledebouriella divaricata*), mint (*Mentha longifolia*) and nut grass (*Cyperus rotundus*), as well as personalized prescriptions from health professionals trained in herbal therapy, which may work even better.[15–19]

How it works: Because of their complexity, herbs have wide-ranging effects throughout the gastrointestinal system, which makes them ideal for the management of IBS where there can be many things amiss. Research has demonstrated that herbal mixtures can reduce pain and act as an anti-spasmodic, reducing muscle spasms and cramps and improving gastrointestinal transit, which may improve diarrhoea and/or constipation, regulate gastric acid production and thus relieve dyspepsia, as well as having anti-inflammatory effects.[20]

Clinical effects: Scientific studies have generally shown that herbal mixtures can offer good symptom relief for some people. Symptoms such as flatulence, sensation of incomplete evacuation, changes in bowel habits (constipation, diarrhoea or both), sensation of tension or fullness, and abdominal pain have all been shown to improve, usually within about four weeks.[21,22] And general quality of life has been shown to improve as well.

Safety: Herbs are generally safe to use long term. Side effects appear to be very rare and may include abdominal cramps, abdominal pain, constipation, diarrhoea, dizziness, nausea and skin rashes. If you are using medication, check with your doctor or a trained herbal medicine practitioner before use. And because the safety of some herbal remedies is unknown, it is best to avoid herbal mixtures altogether if you are pregnant.[23]

Recommended dose: The standard recommended dose of various herbal medicines will vary, but they are usually taken three times a day. A consultation and prescription from a practitioner of herbal medicines is a good idea, or try a quality product from your local health-food store. Follow the label instructions or the advice of your healthcare professional. Herbs may work immediately but typically produce most benefit within two to four weeks of daily use, and improvements increase with time.

Aloe vera

The aloe (*Aloe vera*) plant has triangular gel-filled leaves which have been used as a medicine for thousands of years, first in Egypt and Mesopotamia and now all over the world. Aloe vera gel is made into a juice that is taken internally for digestive health, in particular as a laxative. The Arabic word *alloeh* means 'shining bitter substance' and refers to the bitter, yellow exudate in the green leaf that is responsible for the laxative effect of aloe vera. Aloin is the bitter substance responsible for this effect and when removed by charcoal filtration or hand harvesting, only the gentle, restorative, clear inner-leaf gel remains.

How it works: The clear inner-leaf gel of aloe vera has been shown to reduce gastrointestinal inflammation and has shown preliminary evidence of benefit in people with Inflammatory Bowel Disease.[24] Aloe has also been shown to improve general gastrointestinal health, reducing bad bacteria and bowel putrefaction and improving gastrointestinal motility, digestion and absorption.[25]

Clinical effects: A clinical investigation of aloe vera in people with IBS found that aloe vera improved overall symptoms within one month of treatment. People with diarrhoea-predominant symptoms (IBS-D) responded better to aloe vera, with 43 per cent of people improving with aloe vera versus 22 per cent in the placebo group. Aloe vera reduced pain and improved bowel regularity, in particular.[26] And another study of aloe vera juice found that after eight weeks it significantly reduced abdominal pain and discomfort as well as flatulence in people with constipation-predominant IBS who were not improving with other treatments.[27]

Safety: Clinical studies have found that side effects from aloe vera are no more frequent than placebo, however they include mild nausea or bloating. Aloe vera can also improve blood sugar levels, so speak to your doctor first if you are taking medication for diabetes; otherwise there are no known interactions with medications. And, traditionally, aloe vera is not used during pregnancy, so it should be avoided.

Recommended dose: A dose of 50 ml of juice four times daily has been studied. The aloe juice must be an inner-leaf, aloin-free product so it does not have a laxative effect. Benefits were noticed after one month of use and improvement continued after an additional three months. However, the dose used in a clinical study of people suffering from Inflammatory Bowel Disease is more practical; this study gave 100 ml twice daily, which worked well.

STEP 2: CULTIVATE GOOD BACTERIA

The gut bacteria in people with IBS is distinctly different from people who have healthy digestion and this difference is thought to play an important role in symptoms of abdominal pain and discomfort, changes in bowel habits, bloating and distention, and anxiety or depression.[28] Furthermore, improving the balance of gut bacteria using prebiotics and probiotics has been shown to relieve these symptoms. Step 2 in your Five Steps to Great Gut

Health program is to quickly improve your gut bacteria using prebiotics and/or probiotics, as well as natural foods that boost your beneficial bacteria, so you can improve your symptoms while addressing a major underlying cause of your digestive issues — bad bugs.

Probiotics

The word probiotics comes from the Latin preposition *pro* and the Greek adjective *biotic* literally meaning 'for life'. Probiotics are live bacteria that are consumed as a dietary supplement or in fermented foods such as yoghurt. In 1907 the Nobel laureate Ilya Ilyich Metchnikoff was the first to show that fermented milk containing lactic acid bacteria could change human gut bacteria and have a beneficial health effect. Only in the last few decades, however, has scientific and medical interest in probiotics really taken off and now the use of probiotics is generally accepted in medical practice as an important treatment for some illnesses.

Probiotics have been shown to improve symptoms of IBS, although not all supplements are effective and some are more effective than others for certain symptoms. Below is a guide based on the clinical studies that have shown which probiotics work particularly well and for what symptoms they are most successful.[29-31]

Quick guide to probiotics for symptom relief

Probiotic strain	Typical Dose	Why use this in particular?	How long does it take to work?
Lactobacillus plantarum 299V (DSM 9843)	20 billion CFU daily	Relieves overall symptoms including pain, bloating, incomplete evacuation and flatulence	4 weeks[32–34]
Bifidobacterium infantis 35624	1 billion CFU daily	Relieves overall symptoms including stool frequency, bloating, incomplete evacuation and abdominal pain	4 weeks[35,36]
Multi-strain combination: L. acidophilus CUL60 (NCIMB 30157) and CUL21 (NCIMB 30156), B. lactis CUL34 (NCIMB 30172) and B. bifidum CUL20 (NCIMB 30153)	12.5 to 25 billion CFU daily	Significant improvement in the symptom severity score and in scores for quality of life, days with pain and satisfaction with bowel habit	4 weeks[37]
Escherichia coli DSM 17252	30 drops (providing between 45 to135 million CFU) daily	Relieves overall symptoms including abdominal pain	4–8 weeks[38–40]

Probiotic strain	Typical Dose	Why use this in particular?	How long does it take to work?
Multi-strain blend of eight bacteria: Lactobacillus paracasei, Lactobacillus plantarum, Lactobacillus acidophilus, Lactobacillus delbrueckii (subsp bulgaricus), Bifidobacterium longum, Bifidobacterium breve, Bifidobacterium infantis and Streptococcus thermophilus	450 billion CFU twice daily	May help reduce bloating and flatulence	6–8 weeks[41–43]
Saccharomyces boulardii	10 billion CFU (500 mg) 1-2 times daily	May help reduce diarrhoea or loose, frequent stools	4 weeks[44–47]
Saccharomyces cerevisiae CNCM I-3856	4 billion CFU (500 mg) once daily	May help reduce abdominal pain and discomfort	4 weeks[48]
Bacillus coagulans GBI-30, 6086	2 billion CFU once daily	May help reduce abdominal pain and bloating and reducing diarrhoea or loose, frequent stools	6–8 weeks[49,50]

Note: There is a large variation in dose for probiotics, from tens of millions to almost a trillion CFU (colony forming units, or number of bacteria). This reflects the dose used in the clinical research and is the best guide to ensure efficacy for a particular product. A higher dose does not always mean a product will be more effective. In fact, there is better evidence for lower-dose products. Nor is a multi-strain always better than a single-strain product. It has been suggested that a multi-strain probiotic mixture could be more effective due to a broader spectrum of action than that provided by a single strain. However, current research does not conclusively support this. Evidence that a product is effective, such as a clinical study, is a better guide than the number of different bacteria it provides.[51]

An extra note, on yoghurt: Yoghurt can be made with acidophilus but the types of bacteria used to turn milk into yoghurt are often not the same strains of bacteria shown to have probiotic health effects. And research has shown that yoghurt cultures die off quickly after manufacture and may not influence your gut bacteria at all. Thus, it is incorrect to refer to yoghurt cultures as probiotics unless they have been demonstrated to have a probiotic effect. However, some yoghurts have added probiotics and well established benefits. Look for yoghurts with added probiotic strains; these will normally be stated in the nutrition information on the label. But beware the 'health halo' — just because a food has added probiotics does not mean it's healthy.[52,53]

If you are going to use a probiotic follow the recommended dose on the product label or the advice from your practitioner and take it daily for a minimum of four weeks to see if you improve. If you do benefit you can continue the probiotic long term if necessary. If one probiotic does not improve your symptoms, trial a different product to see if that works better for you.[54]

The probiotic strains listed above have good evidence that they can improve symptoms, and they are generally not difficult to find and purchase in most countries. If you are considering using a different probiotic supplement, ask the manufacturer if there have been any studies showing that it works. However, it is possible a probiotic not mentioned on this list or that has not been studied will still work perfectly well for you, so you can still consider trying different products.

Safety: Probiotic supplements are generally considered very safe, with rare and mild side effects that are not significantly different from placebo. Some probiotics have been shown to make symptoms worse, so it is important to use a product that has been scientifically studied. Probiotics are sometimes added to yoghurt, which is fine, but you should avoid these if you have dairy intolerance. Probiotics can be used safely alongside medications and are also considered safe for use during pregnancy.

Prebiotics

In 1978, Japanese researchers were the first to show that special types of dietary fibres were able to beneficially change the bacterial ecosystem in the gut.[55] These special types of fibres are called prebiotics and are unique in that, although we do not digest them and use them for energy, our good bifidobacteria do. Bifidobacteria use prebiotics to grow and increase in number, which has wide-ranging benefits for digestive and general health.

Because bifidobacteria play a host of important roles in maintaining digestive health, and low levels of bifidobacteria are common in people with symptoms of IBS, prebiotics are a particularly promising therapy. Experimental evidence suggests prebiotics may counter a number of the underlying features of

IBS, including changes in gastrointestinal transit time, pain hypersensitivity, small intestinal bacterial overgrowth (SIBO), and excessive fermentation and gas. The results of two clinical studies have found that prebiotics can significantly improve digestive symptoms.[56–58]

Quick guide to prebiotics for symptom relief

Prebiotic	Why use this in particular?	How much should I take?	How long does it take to work?
Galacto-oligosaccharides	Improved overall symptoms including stool consistency, flatulence and bloating.	3.5 g daily	Up to 4 weeks
Short-chain fructo-oligosaccharides	Reduces incidence and intensity of symptoms including bloating, pain, straining and incomplete bowel movements.	5 g daily	Up to 6 weeks

It is important to follow the recommended dosage, as higher doses may make symptoms worse; the dosages above, however, are unlikely to cause problems. There are many other prebiotics available (e.g. inulin, long-chain fructo-oligosaccharides and various fibre blends) and you could try these at a dose of no more than 5 g daily to see if they help. But keep in mind these have not been well studied and may not work or could even make your symptoms worse.

Safety: During the first few days of taking prebiotics, increases in gastrointestinal symptoms are common with diarrhoea, flatulence, abdominal pain and nausea the most frequent. If you do get an increase in symptoms, and they are mild, continue treatment for a few days to see if they pass, and they usually do, but if not, it may be best to stop treatment and try a probiotic instead. If you have a dairy sensitivity it would be best not to use trans-galacto-oligosaccharides, as these are derived from milk. Prebiotics can be used safely alongside medications and are also considered safe for use during pregnancy.

Natural foods

Healthy food is good for you and your gut bacteria. For example, diets high in calories, refined sugars, fat and protein (typically from processed foods, sweets and high-fat animal products) increase levels of bad bacteria in the gut, while diets rich in complex carbohydrates (from wholegrains, fruits and vegetables) not only lower levels of bad bugs but increase your levels of healthy bifidobacteria too.[59] In addition to generally eating well, a number of foods have been shown to have natural bifidobacteria-boosting effects.

Apples: Eating two apples daily significantly increased bifidobacteria within just seven days, and other beneficial bacteria such as lactobacillus also tended to increase as well.[60] However, apples can upset some people and are best avoided initially.

Bananas: In one study, women who ate a banana twice daily as a pre-meal snack for two months had a slight increase in good bifidobacteria levels and a significant reduction in bloating. In fact, before the study, they were bloated almost every day but adding bananas to their diet cut their symptoms in half.[61]

Blueberries: Blueberries are very high in polyphenols which, like fibre, act as a prebiotic and boost your good gut bacteria. Consuming a wild blueberry drink equivalent to approximately 175 g of fresh blueberries doubled bifidobacteria in the gut after six weeks.[62] Dark-skinned grapes may have a similar effect.[63]

Cocoa: Like blueberries, cocoa is very high in polyphenols and has a natural prebiotic effect. A dark chocolate drink each day for four weeks was able to significantly increase bifidobacteria and lactobacillus in the gut and decrease potentially harmful clostridium bacteria.[64]

Green tea: Packed full of polyphenols, green tea can boost your bacteria too. Drinking about 4 cups of green tea daily balanced out gut bacteria within 10 days, increasing the relative proportion of bifidobacteria.[65]

Wholegrains: Wholegrains are higher in fibre and therefore more likely to improve your gut bacteria. Studies have found that eating a wholegrain breakfast cereal daily, results in a significant increase in bifidobacteria compared to a non-wholegrain cereal.[66,67]

So look after your bacteria, and yourself, and consume some of these healthy foods regularly. An advantage over prebiotic supplements is that foods are relatively cheap, completely natural, they taste great, and are unlikely to make your symptoms worse, apart from wholegrain wheat perhaps. You could try using a prebiotic in the short term while you start to include more of these foods in your regular diet. Keep in mind that, although these foods are beneficial, they have not specifically been shown to improve digestive symptoms, so probiotics and prebiotics are a surer way to get relief.

STEP 3: CALM DOWN YOUR NERVOUS GUT

Because your central nervous system directly influences your gastrointestinal function, your mood and the way you deal with stress can contribute to your digestive symptoms. And, importantly, having digestive problems is in itself stressful and living with symptoms can place a great deal of pressure on you — your gastrointestinal ill health can trigger your stress response and affect your emotions and ability to cope. Relaxation and mind–body therapies can help you break the stress cycle and improve emotional and gastrointestinal symptoms as well as your overall quality of life.

Step 3 of your Five Steps to Great Gut Health is to reduce the stress in your gut and nervous system by learning three very simple and effective techniques that will help you relax and reduce physical tension:

- using abdominal breathing to quickly produce a relaxation response in your nervous system to reduce stress and improve digestion
- practising meditation to help diminish emotional and physical symptoms of stress long term
- keeping a daily diary to help you identify and respond more effectively to situations that may be causing you trouble.

Recognizing how stress affects you, and how you respond to it, can help you develop more flexible ways of managing your symptoms.[68]

1. Abdominal breathing

Abdominal breathing, also known as diaphragmatic breathing, is a powerful way to decrease stress by activating the relaxation response in your nervous system. This technique is a simple and quick way to place your body and mind in a state of relaxation and over time may reduce tension and fatigue. Initially, practise this technique three times daily for 10–15 minutes before meals, then after one month you can reduce it to just one to two times a day if you like. To begin:

- Find a comfortable place to sit or lie down, with your feet slightly apart, one hand on your abdomen near the navel, and the other hand on your chest.
- Gently exhale the air in your lungs through your mouth, and then inhale slowly through your nose to the count of four, pushing out your abdomen slightly and concentrating on your breath. As you breathe in, imagine warm air flowing all over your body. Hold the breath for a count of at least four but not more than seven.
- Slowly exhale through your mouth while counting to eight. Gently contract your abdominal muscles to completely release the remaining air in the lungs.
- Repeat until you feel deeply relaxed for a total of five cycles. You may be able to do only one or two cycles at first.

Once you feel comfortable with your ability to breathe into the abdomen, it is not necessary to use your hands on your abdomen and chest.

2. Meditate daily

Regular practice of meditation can increase physical and mental relaxation, reduce stress and improve emotional stability.[69] Meditation has been shown to promote relaxed brainwave activity, enhance cognitive function and reduce the emotional and physical symptoms of stress.[70] Try the following simple meditation exercise. Practise it once a day; in the morning or late evening generally works best, or any time you will be uninterrupted for a few minutes. To begin:

- Sit in a comfortable position. Try to sit in the same place each day and avoid positions that you might fall asleep in. When in position, your back should be long and support itself; your shoulders should be relaxed downward, your neck long, and your chin pointing neither up nor down; and your face should be relaxed.

- Begin to breathe (preferably through your nostrils). Feel your belly rise, your ribs expand, and the slight movement in your collarbones and shoulders as the breath moves upward. Feel the exhalation.

- Focus on one aspect of the breath: the movement of air in and out of your nostrils; the lifting and falling of your belly; and think about that one aspect of the breath. When your mind wanders, gently bring it back to the breath and the aspect you have chosen to watch. Do this as many times as you need to. There is no such thing as a good or bad meditation ('good' and 'bad' are judgments — just note them and go back to the breathing).

Start with 5–10 minutes and then increase the time until you can sit for 30 minutes.

3. Record and reflect

When you have chronic digestive problems it is sometimes difficult to objectively reflect on how bad your symptoms are each day, and how different events and situations affect the severity of your gastrointestinal complaints. To give you a clearer picture on how your symptoms vary and to help you identify stressful events that might be playing a role, you can use Your Daily Symptom Diary, opposite. Create your own diary in a ruled notebook and fill it in each day as best you can for three months.

At the end of every day, fill out the diary rating of each individual symptom on a scale of 1 to 10, 1 being very mild and 10 being very severe. Include any medications or natural supplements you might use for acute symptom relief. You can also fill this in each morning for the previous day if that is more convenient.

On the opposite page of your notebook, answer each of the following questions in order each day:

- Did you experience a stressful event today?
- What was the event?
- How did you feel emotionally in that situation?
- What were your physical sensations while it was happening?
- Did you notice any change in your symptoms while it was happening?

At the end of each week, see if there is a relationship between the score in Your Daily Symptom Diary and your answers to these questions. This will help you identify situations or events that may be exacerbating your symptoms and enable you to take steps towards changing them or improving how you react or respond to them.

Your Daily Symptom Diary

	Pain, cramps or discomfort	Loose stools, sudden urges, or diarrhoea	Straining or constipation	Bloating or distention	Excessive flatulence	Anxiety, and/ or depression	Fatigue or tiredness
Mon							
Tues							
Wed							
Thur							
Fri							
Sat							
Sun							

Scale: 0 None — 1 — 2 — 3 Mild — 4 — 5 Moderate — 6 — 7 — 8 Strong — 9 — 10 Severe

STEP 4: PUT YOUR DIGESTION ON A DIET

Your food plan is a simple way to swiftly reduce your exposure to potentially problematic foods and ease your symptoms. The plan then involves slowly reintroducing common problem foods to see if they are, indeed, a cause of your problems. Because a modern processed diet may be linked to the development of digestive symptoms, the plan is also a template for healthy eating, so think of this as a way to quickly reduce symptoms and identify food intolerances to fast-track you towards long-term healthy eating for improved digestion.

Some of the key ways the diet works:

- eliminates common problem foods, then tests them so you know what they are
- reduces your exposure to artificial additives and foods that can disrupt your gut bacteria
- reduces your intake of sugar and carbohydrates that feed bad bugs
- increases intake and abundance of foods that improve gut bacteria, diversity and health
- provides a simple guide to methods that can help reduce symptoms, including a regular meal pattern; avoidance of large meals; and reduced intake of fat, insoluble fibres, caffeine and gas-producing foods such as beans, cabbage, and onions
- it is a modified and more manageable version of diets reviewed in this book including the Specific Carbohydrate Diet (SCD) and the low-FODMAP diet.

Initially you will eliminate major problem foods, such as gluten and lactose, during a clear-out period; the aim is to reduce your exposure to foods that could be triggering your symptoms and to give your digestive system a break. After four weeks you will reintroduce the major problem foods one by one to see if they are triggering your symptoms. This method is called an elimination and re-challenge diet and is a well established and effective way to identify food intolerances.

In addition to eliminating potential food intolerances, your food plan will reduce your intake of generally unhealthy foods. A typical modern diet — high in processed foods, fatty meats, high-fat dairy products, sugars, refined grains and additives, and low in fruits, vegetables, wholegrains, legumes, nuts, fish and lean meats — could be contributing to your illness, so eating a healthy diet is an important part of reducing your symptoms. The only side effects are likely to be losing excess weight, feeling better and reducing your risk of other diet-related diseases. The diet plan is divided into two phases: Phase 1: Clear out and clean up and Phase 2: Eat and evaluate.

Phase 1: Clear out and clean up

Phase 1 is a four-week plan based on five guiding rules to *clear out* major problem foods including gluten, dairy, lactose, high-carbohydrate and high-fat foods and to *clean up* your diet in general, making sure it is nutritionally balanced and super healthy. This phase is restrictive and will take careful planning and preparation, so think through what you are going to eat each day and shop judiciously. You will need to be particularly mindful when you know you will be eating away from home as well, so plan ahead or pack your own food. It is important to eat only the recommended foods in the following tables. Remember, once you have finished Phase 2 you will be able to eat more freely again.

Rule 1: Eat lean protein foods at most meals

Try to include lean protein-rich foods regularly (one to two times daily). Animal foods are an important source of dietary fat which can aggravate your symptoms, which is why it is very important to choose lean cuts. And protein can be fermented by bad bacteria, which is why some people find that protein-rich foods can aggravate symptoms, so you may need to find a level that works for you.[71]

As you embark on your dietary change it is a good idea to start recording what you eat each day in a food diary: keep a notebook and take five minutes to record what you have eaten. This simple practice will help you to plan and reflect on your experience, and help you make the initial changes. After a month or so, you will find you no longer need the food diary.

LEAN PROTEIN FOODS (Average serving size = 90–100 g cooked)
PHASE 1
Fish, shellfish Lamb, lean Poultry: chicken (breast only), turkey Beef, very lean Pork, lean
ALLOWED AFTER PHASE 2
Soy or veggie burger Fat-free yoghurt, plain Cottage cheese, non-fat or low-fat Low-fat yoghurt, plain Ricotta, part skim or non-fat (3–4 tablespoons) Tofu (200 g) Eggs (2 whole) Tempeh Mozzarella, part skim or non-fat (60 g)

The foods permitted only in Phase 2 are common problem foods; soy and veggie burgers may contain gluten or grains and dairy foods may contain too much lactose. Include these after you have tested for food intolerances as part of Phase 2.

When choosing protein-rich foods, avoid processed meats such as bacon, salami and pepperoni, as these contain nitrates which produce toxic compounds in your gut and may have negative long-term health effects.

It is important to choose lean cuts of meat, as a high intake of saturated fat may contribute to bloating, distention, pain and diarrhoea. Organic, free-range (meats, poultry, soy, dairy and eggs), grass-fed (meats) and non-farmed (fish) choices are healthier.

Rule 2: Consume plenty of vegetables and a little fruit

Vegetables and fruits are a very important part of a healthy diet, however certain vegetables and fruits are best avoided for the first four weeks of your food plan as they can aggravate symptoms. You can consume vegetables more freely after Phase 2. Aim for one serving two to three times daily.

VEGETABLES (Average serving size = 1 coffee mug or 50% of your plate cooked or raw)	
PHASE 1	
Alfalfa	Fennel*
Eggplant (aubergine)	Green beans
Bean sprouts	Bamboo shoots

VEGETABLES
(Average serving size = 1 coffee mug or 50% of your plate cooked or raw)

PHASE 1

Lettuce/mixed greens: cos (romaine), red and green leaf varieties, endive (chicory), spinach, rocket (arugula), radicchio, watercress	Greens: bok choy, Swiss chard (silver beet), kale, spinach, mustard, or beet greens (the leaves and stalks of beetroot)
Capsicum (bell or other peppers)	Snow peas (mangetout)*
Broccoli*	Peas*
Brussels sprouts*	Radishes
Cabbage (all types)	Salsa (sugar-free)
Celery	Sea vegetables (kelp, etc.)
Zucchinis (courgettes)	Sugar snap peas*
Cucumber	Tomatoes
Chives	Water chestnuts

ALLOWED AFTER PHASE 2

Artichokes	Chicory
Asparagus	Mushrooms
Onion, leeks, shallots, garlic, scallions	Okra
Cauliflower	

The vegetables permitted only in Phase 2 may be too high in prebiotic fibres, which can ferment and aggravate your symptoms, so include these after you have tested for food intolerances. Foods marked with an asterisk (*) can be consumed up to half a cup raw or cooked per day.

You can also include a variety of herbs, spices and condiments during Phases 1 and 2 including cinnamon, mustard, tamari soy sauce, vinegar, lime juice, lemon juice, fresh or dried herbs, pepper, garlic-infused olive oil, fresh or dried chilli and ginger.

Fruits are also a very important part of a healthy diet but, like vegetables, some fruits could be aggravating your symptoms so are best avoided initially. Aim for two servings of fruits daily, but not more than this. Serving sizes are provided below.

FRUIT (Average serving size as indicated below)	
PHASE 1	
Apricots (3 medium)	Passionfruit (3)
Banana (1 medium)	Pawpaw/papaya (½ medium)
Berries: blackberries, blueberries, raspberries, cranberries, strawberries (1 handful = 80 g)	Pineapple (½ cup)
Grapes (15)	Orange (1 large)
Rockmelon (cantaloupe) (½ medium)	Peaches, yellow (2 small)
Grapefruit (1 whole)	Tangerines (2 small)

FRUIT (Average serving size as indicated below)	
PHASE 1	
Honeydew melon (½ medium)	
Kiwifruit (2–3)	
ALLOWED AFTER PHASE 2	
Apple (1 medium)	Persimmon (1 medium)
Pear (1 medium)	Peaches, white (2 small)
Mango (½ medium)	Watermelon (2 handfuls chopped)
Nectarines (2 small)	Cherries (15)
Plums (2 small)	Fresh figs (2)

The fruits permitted only in Phase 2 may contain too much fructose or prebiotic fibres, which can aggravate symptoms for some people. Include these after you have tested for food intolerances.

It is important to avoid dry and tinned fruits, as these are especially concentrated sources of both natural and added sugars.

Rule 3: Include good fats in your diet

Good fats are those found in foods such as fish, nuts, seeds and cold-pressed vegetable oils. These dietary fats are especially good for your heart, skin, immune system, brain and digestive system. However, because fatty meals may aggravate your symptoms, even those containing good fats, it is important to limit your intake to a healthy level. As a rule, enjoy some nuts, nut butter and seeds daily (aim for one serving daily, which is about a handful). Walnuts and almonds are particularly healthy choices (cashews and pistachios are high in fermentable fibres so are not recommended; however, you could reintroduce these slowly after Phase 2). Use only healthy oils: for cooking, cold-pressed extra virgin olive oil is best; and for salads cold-pressed olive, walnut or flaxseed (linseed) oils are ideal. Store salad oils in a cool, dark place or keep refrigerated. Try not to exceed two servings daily. The following list will ensure you get the right amount of good fats in your diet.

NUTS AND SEEDS (Average serving size as indicated)	
Almonds or hazelnuts (10–12 whole nuts)	Pistachios, sunflower, pumpkin (pepita) or sesame seeds (2 tablespoons)
Walnut or pecan halves (7–8)	Nut butter (1 tablespoon made from the above nuts)
Peanuts (18 nuts or 2 tablespoons)	Pine nuts (2 tablespoons)

HEALTHY OILS Average serving size = 1 tablespoon (3 teaspoons) or as indicated	
Avocado (⅛)	Mayonnaise (from canola oil)
Flaxseed/linseed oil (refrigerate)	Olives (8–10 medium)
Extra virgin olive oil (preferable), coconut oil and canola (rapeseed) oil for cooking	Walnut oil (refrigerate) Hemp oil (refrigerate)

Rule 4: Limit carbohydrate-rich foods

High-carbohydrate diets have been linked to digestive symptoms, and people tend to improve when they reduce their intake of these foods, which include breads, pastries, cakes, biscuits, pasta, cereals, beans, legumes, potato, soft drinks (sodas), desserts and confectionery. Reducing your intake might be difficult at first as people often base the majority of their diet on these foods, but it will get easier and become natural with time.

Aim for two servings daily of the recommended foods below, only one of which should be grains such as rice, quinoa or bread. At least one serving, or both, should be carbohydrate-rich vegetables like pumpkin or carrots.

CARBOHYDRATE-RICH FOODS (Average serving size = ½ cup cooked or as indicated)	
PHASE 1	
Amaranth	Bread: gluten free (2 slices)
Rice: Basmati, brown rice, wild rice	Carrots (½ cup cooked or 2 medium raw)

Buckwheat	Parsnip
Corn flour, polenta	Potato
Swede	Pumpkin (squash)
Oats: rolled oats, oatcakes (2 each)	Quinoa
Butternut squash/pumpkin	Sweet potato (½ medium, baked)
Millet	Turnip
ALLOWED AFTER PHASE 2	
Barley	Hummus (50 g or 4 tablespoons)
Beetroot	Wheat: wholegrain wheat crackers (3 each), 100% whole wheat bread (1–2 slices)
Bulgur (cracked wheat)	Rye: wholegrain wheat crackers (3 each), 100% whole rye bread (1–2 slices)
Bean soups (175 ml)	Spelt: 100% whole spelt bread (1–2 slices)
Sweet corn (½ cob)	Split peas, sweet green peas, lentils, garden peas (3 tablespoons)
Beans: chickpeas (garbanzo beans), pinto, kidney, black, lima, cannellini, navy, mung beans, fat-free refried, green, soybeans (3 tablespoons)	

The carbohydrate-rich foods permitted only in Phase 2 include bulgur, barley, spelt, rye and wheat, which contain gluten. People who are gluten sensitive do not always tolerate oats, even if they are labelled as gluten free, so you might want to eliminate these initially as well. Legumes, beans, peas, beetroot and corn are high in prebiotic fibres or fructose, which may aggravate your symptoms.

If you suspect you have coeliac disease or are sensitive to gluten you must get a medical test before you eliminate gluten from your diet. If you eliminate gluten now, the test results may falsely show up negative (not coeliac) because you are no longer exposed to gluten.

Rule 5: Drink mostly water

Regular consumption of drinks containing sugars such as milk, fruit juice and soft drinks (sodas) could be aggravating your digestive symptoms because of their high sugar content. For this reason it is important to avoid these and drink mainly water or herbal teas. Aim to drink about 2 litres (8 glasses) of filtered water each day including any teas or coffee.

DRINKS AND BEVERAGES Average daily serving size = as indicated	
Purified water (approx. 8 glasses)	Herbal teas (2–3 cups)
Green tea (2–3 cups)	Rice or almond milk, unsweetened (150 ml)
Black tea (1–2 cups)	
ALLOWED AFTER PHASE 2	
Milk, skimmed or semi-skimmed, lactose free (150 ml)	Fresh fruit juices (1 glass)

Soda water (1 glass)	Coffee substitutes (1 cup)
Coffee (1–2 cups)	Soy milk, plain, unsweetened (150 ml)

The drinks and beverages permitted only in Phase 2 are concentrated sources of sugars such as fructose and lactose, which can be a cause of digestive symptoms for some people. Coffee substitutes including dandelion root may contain gluten, lactose or prebiotic fibre. Include these after you have tested for food intolerances.

Avoid soft drinks (sodas), diet soft drinks (diet sodas), cordials, sweetened fruit juices, vitamin water and sports drinks completely; apart from potentially causing digestive issues due to their sugar or artificial sweetener content, they are generally unhealthy.

If you do drink alcohol, keep within healthy drinking guidelines or no more than one to two standard drinks daily, as more than this can aggravate IBS symptoms.[72]

If you drink one or more cups of coffee daily, reduce slowly over the first one to two weeks, as suddenly stopping can cause headaches and mood changes.

If you use sweeteners avoid fructose, agave syrup and xylitol and use either plain table sugar or maple syrup.

Phase 2: Eat and evaluate

After the initial four weeks of Phase 1 you now *eat* and challenge problem foods and *evaluate* any possible food intolerances by carefully paying attention to any increase in symptoms.

After following Phase 1 of your diet for four weeks you can start to reintroduce potential problem foods to see if they make your symptoms worse. This requires reintroducing suspect foods and carefully noting any symptoms over the following days. Any new, returning or increase in symptoms is likely to be attributable to that food. The food is then removed from your diet to see if symptoms clear again.

If you have tested positive for a food intolerance already by one of the methods described in the previous chapters, you do not need to perform a challenge. You can also skip the challenge if you already avoid a food because it causes you problems. It typically takes 30 days to complete Phase 2, fewer if you are not testing all the listed foods.

How Phase 2 works:

Reintroduce one new food group every three days (see guide on the following page).

At least three servings of the food need to be eaten on the challenge day, at two to three separate meals.

After the challenge day, return to the Phase 1 diet for two days, and take note of any changes to your symptoms.

If your symptoms get worse on the challenge days, don't consume any more, and return to the Phase 1 diet until symptoms have resolved before moving on to the next challenge.

Challenge foods that cause no symptoms are not incorporated back into the diet until all challenges are completed.

Challenge foods need to be challenged individually (e.g. when challenging wheat, don't serve it with cheese).

Keep a record of the food challenge, including what you ate and the time you ate it, in your symptoms diary (page 183). Continue to record your digestive symptoms and note any changes in symptoms during the challenge (three days) and afterwards (two days).

Challenge	One serving is equivalent to
Lactose/Dairy	1 glass (250 ml/1 cup) milk
Gluten/Wheat	2 slices of wholemeal wheat bread
Fructose	1 glass (250 ml/1 cup) apple juice
Coffee	1 strong cup black coffee
Eggs	1 egg
Soy	1 glass (250 ml/1 cup) unsweetened soy milk

Testing for lactose and fructose intolerance with a breath test (see pages 119 and 135) is preferable and if you have done this you can skip these food challenges. Coeliac disease can only be confirmed with a medical test (page 119). If you have been diagnosed with coeliac disease skip this challenge also. However, you may have non-coeliac gluten sensitivity in which case a food challenge is an ideal way to identify whether or not gluten is a problem.

If you are not sensitive to any of the foods, the process was not a waste of time. At least you know the foods are not a problem!

If you do find you are sensitive to any of the challenge foods above, it does not mean you have to eliminate them completely; rather, you may find your symptoms improve when you reduce consumption to a certain level. People with lactose intolerance can still eat dairy and tolerate small amounts of lactose, and people who are fructose intolerant can still eat foods containing some fructose. You may also find your tolerance improves over time.

Coffee, soy or eggs are relatively simple foods to minimize or avoid if you find you have an intolerance; however if you find lactose, fructose or gluten are problem foods you will need to enlist the help of an experienced nutrition professional to help you develop a dietary plan that reduces or eliminates your exposure while ensuring your diet remains nutritionally balanced.

Once you have finished testing for food intolerances you can start to slowly bring more foods back into your diet — mainly the foods in the tables listed under ALLOWED AFTER PHASE 2, provided you do not have an intolerance to them. Just be mindful of any increase in symptoms attributable to a food. And by now you will have a good feel for what foods and serving sizes you should be aiming for each day moving forward with your new healthy way of eating.

STEP 5: STAY SYMPTOM-FREE FOR LIFE

The reason you developed digestive symptoms is most likely your unique susceptibility to digestive disease, so you may find that for you it is important to develop and maintain some general lifestyle practices that keep your symptoms at bay and prevent them from flaring up again, even if you have managed to reduce or completely relieve them.

Here are five general recommendations that you could incorporate into your daily life that may help optimize your digestive health in the long term. They are also important for preventing a lot of other diet- and lifestyle-related diseases and improving your overall wellbeing. These are general guiding principles, so feel free to interpret and adopt these in ways that suit your own way of life.

Eat well

Maintaining a healthy, balanced diet that emphasizes fruits, vegetables, nuts, seeds, legumes, wholegrains, lean meats and fish is important for maintaining your digestive health. The food plan in this book is an excellent template for a highly nutritious, minimally processed, natural diet designed to keep you and your digestion healthy. In addition, try to buy organic whenever possible.

While the devastating effects of a Western diet on heart disease, type 2 diabetes and obesity are well known, less attention has been paid to the link between food and digestive illness. As we have explored in this book, high-fat, high-carbohydrate, unhealthy modern diets could be linked to the development of IBS, so healthy eating should be part of your long-term strategy to stay well.

Nevertheless, most people know what they should eat to keep well; the trick is making lifestyle changes that make healthy eating an unconscious part of your life, not a daily battle. A good way to do this is to adopt some simple rules:

- When you shop, do not buy food you shouldn't eat.
- Try a new healthy recipe each week.
- Do not eat with the television on.
- Pack healthy lunches each morning.
- Eat fruit or nuts as a snack.
- Use 25 cm (10 in) plates for dinner.
- Cover 50 per cent of your plate with vegetables.

While we may think we have conscious control over what we eat, a large and grossly underestimated determinant of our eating behaviour is environmental cues such as package size, plate shape, lighting, odours, variety, proximity, convenience and sight.

'Every single one of us is influenced by what's around us when it comes to deciding what and when we will eat,' says Professor Brian Wansink, author of *Mindless Eating: Why we eat more than we think*. Many of our food choices, it seems, are actually beyond our conscious awareness. Simple rules of thumb can 'take your mind off the game' and turn mindless eating into mindlessly eating better.

In addition to healthy eating, a good-quality multivitamin and mineral supplement containing additional vitamin D, and an omega-3 fatty acid supplement is a relatively cheap and very safe way to ensure optimal nutrition and they could play an important role in reducing and preventing symptoms. Vitamin D supplementation, for example, has been shown to help reduce symptoms in people with IBS and other digestive illnesses.[73]

Exercise most days

Most health recommendations suggest you should aim for a minimum of 30 minutes of light to moderate exercise, such as brisk walking, most days of the week. However, most people are not even reaching this modest amount. Daily physical activity is a crucial part of a healthy lifestyle and needs to become part of your daily life in a way that is realistic, manageable and enjoyable.

Physical activity has a profound effect on your health, which is why regular exercise can improve and reduce the risk of so many diseases — obesity, heart disease, type 2 diabetes, hypertension, stroke, breast cancer, colon cancer, osteoporosis, depression, anxiety and a decline in cognitive performance in older age. Regular exercise will also keep your digestive system functioning well and help you deal with stress more successfully — two major reasons why staying active may help stave off digestive symptoms, especially bloating and constipation.

Instead of hearing more about how good it is for you to be active, you need to build regular exercise into your daily life. Often people say that they have no time for activity but you *can* make time; it is more likely that exercise is simply a low priority in your day. Building daily habits into your life like a morning walk for a paper, a midday swim, an afternoon walk with a friend, or setting up a treadmill in front of the TV in the evening, are easy solutions. And you could take up any number of active pastimes — the gym, fitness classes, walking groups, yoga, jogging, swimming or cycling, for example. Just find things you enjoy.

Cultivate resilience

Virtually everyone today lives with some form of chronic stress, which may be why stress-related illnesses such as chronic fatigue, depression, anxiety and IBS are so common. There are many different ways to minimize the negative effects stress can have on your digestion and overall health. Advice on how to reduce stress often centres on techniques such as meditation and yoga, and while these can reduce physical and emotional tension, there are other important determinants of your ability to handle stress that are more important but receive less attention, such as a sense of family, social connection, community and belonging.

Professor Andrew Steptoe from the University College London and his colleagues have been investigating the protective effect of positive emotions such as happiness, joy, excitement, enthusiasm, and contentment on physical health. They have found that people who experience higher levels of these emotions are much less likely to suffer from disease. Importantly, what they have also found is that happier people do not experience less stress and adversity in their lives but rather they have more social support, a higher level of social connectedness and are more likely to be optimistic. Social connection gives you access to protective resources that enable you to handle problems flexibly and more effectively.

So minimizing stress, or 'stress management', is not the only solution; we all face stress but we do not all succumb to it, and what you need to do is 'cultivate resilience'. The ways in which you can do this are to develop a healthy lifestyle, because your ability to cope with stress is dependent on, and improved by, a wide variety of factors including social connection, time with family and friends, work–life balance, regular holidays, time spent in nature, healthy eating, physical activity, a good night's sleep, a sense of purpose, an optimistic outlook, spiritual practice and mind–body therapies such as meditation and yoga. These are all important ways to improve your ability to deal with stress and cultivate resilience.

Get a good night's sleep

Sleep is essential for restoring health and vitality to your mind and body each day. Studies show that people who sleep seven to eight hours each night live longer, healthier lives than those who sleep fewer hours. A single good night's rest can reduce the severity of digestive symptoms and, conversely, poor sleep could actually be a major cause of symptoms for some people. Prioritizing a good night's sleep is a simple but powerful way to preserve optimal health.

Being more mindful about the importance of a good night's sleep and developing healthy sleeping habits will ensure you get adequate sleep each day. Here are some healthy sleep habits:

- Avoid caffeinated drinks such as coffee and tea, especially late in the day.
- Avoid exercise four hours before bedtime — although daily exercise promotes good sleep, exercise shortly before bedtime could hinder your sleep.
- Avoid daytime naps, as they can disrupt your body clock.
- Go to bed at the same time each day, even if you are not particularly tired, and try to get out of bed at a regular time too.
- Turn your bedroom into a sleep sanctuary — soften the colours and lights; fit heavy blinds on the windows so it is as dark as possible; keep the room at a comfortable temperature; do not read, watch TV or use a computer; and leave your phone out of your bedroom.
- Regularly schedule relaxation time before bed (e.g. aromatherapy, listening to relaxing music or taking a warm bath).
- Use earplugs if noise is a problem.
- Try to get exposure to daytime light for at least 30 minutes in the morning to help regulate your body clock.

Beyond keeping your digestive system well, you will find regular good-quality sleep has countless health benefits including boosting your mood, energy and overall wellbeing.

Self-medicate, naturally

Humans have been self-medicating with natural medicines for thousands of years. Over 100 years before probiotics became popular, the health benefits of fermented foods were known, and herbal medicines have a written history dating back 5000 years. Chances are we have been suffering digestive problems and treating them with natural medicines as long as we have been human.

Identifying and dealing with the fundamental cause of the problem has been the focus of this book, and hopefully you have been able to work out what the major issues are for you to improve or completely resolve your symptoms. However, there is a chance a symptom will continue or reappear, in which case you may want to consider treatment with some of the natural medicines described in this book.

One of the most characteristic underlying problems with IBS is a change in your gut bacteria, and it is for this reason probiotics can be tremendously helpful. If you have found that a probiotic has worked well for you, there is no apparent harm in continuing to take it long term to keep your digestive system well. Give it a rest now and then to see if your symptoms are fine without it, and don't worry about skipping a few days between doses, as the benefits tend not to be affected too quickly.

You could also take digestive enzymes with meals you know cause problems. For some people this strategy has been found to keep symptoms at bay for years. And occasional use of the herbal medicines mentioned in Step 1: Get fast symptom relief (page 161) would be appropriate if your symptoms flare up. They are generally very safe and good to have on hand in your natural-medicine cupboard.

THE ROAD TO REGAINING YOUR DIGESTIVE HEALTH

Throughout this book we have taken a journey through several underappreciated but important reasons why things may be out of balance in the digestive system, including a wide range of dietary and lifestyle factors. Because we live in a pill-popping culture, we frequently believe that medicines, including natural ones, may be the answer, however it's only when we understand the bigger picture that true healing can begin.

The purpose of this book has been to explore that bigger picture and understand how things such as our environment, sleep, stress, physical activity, nutrition and diet can work in profound and very personal ways to influence our health. While these determinants of digestive health may seem straightforward, it is often simple lifestyle changes that are the most powerful medicine — that is, *knowing* what is going to work for you. With the knowledge laid out in these pages it is now possible for you to regain your digestive health, which will in turn extend to improvements in the vitality of your mind and body and enable you to live a happier, healthier life.

ACKNOWLEDGMENTS

Over the last decade or so while immersed in clinical practice, research and teaching integrative medicine, I have made a few attempts to author a book, and I am glad I did not until now. Although I am not deterministic, I believe this book came together at the perfect time: a serendipitous mixture of authentic motivation, enough experience to bring maturity and perspective, combined with the support of the wonderful people who believed in me.

Along the road I have been blessed to have worked and developed friendships with colleagues who have inspired me, shaped my thinking and grounded me in the traditions and practice of natural medicine. These notably include Jeff Bland PhD and Deanna Minich PhD of the Personalized Lifestyle Medicine Institute, both of whom have been deeply inspirational. Few people have been as great a catalyst for positive change in health care as Jeff. I am also greatly inspired by the many naturopathic physicians who are helping to establish the science and clinical practice of naturopathic medicine including Jonathan Prousky ND, editor of the *Journal of Orthomolecular Medicine* and author and researcher Alan Logan ND. The motivation may have been small but the effect was exponential, thank you. And to my close friends Hannah Yang ND, Debbie Cotton ND, Aliza Marogy NT and Nigma Talib ND, thank you for your feedback, encouragement and the countless hours of 'naturopathic conversation'. Dr Brown's book is finally here.

I would also like to thank the team at Exisle Publishing for the opportunity to bring this work to the countless people it has the potential to help. I am deeply grateful and had to pinch myself at first. A special thank you to Anouska Jones for seeing the promise of the book and to Monica Berton for her beautiful work on the manuscript.

Finally, I would like to acknowledge the unconditional love of my mother and father, whose support from the beginning of my naturopathic studies along the sometimes rocky road to where I am today has been unwavering. Thank you beyond words.

RESOURCES

Integrative health professionals

American Association of Naturopathic Physicians: www.naturopathic.org

Australian Traditional Medicine Society Ltd: www.atms.com.au

British Association for Applied Nutrition and Nutritional Therapy (BANT): www.bant.org.uk

Canadian Association of Naturopathic Doctors: www.cand.ca

Complementary and Natural Healthcare Council (United Kingdom): www.cnhc.org.uk

Institute for Functional Medicine (global): www.functionalmedicine.org

Books

Hunter, J, *Irritable Bowel Solutions: The essential guide to irritable bowel syndrome, its causes and treatments*, Random House, UK, 2007.

Hunter, J, *Solve Your Food Intolerance: A practical dietary programme to eliminate food intolerance*, (rev. edn), Vermilion, London, 2005.

Lackner, J, *Controlling IBS the Drug-free Way: A 10-step plan for symptom relief*, Stewart, Tabori and Chang, New York, 2007.

Shepherd, S and Gibson, P, *The Complete Low-FODMAP Diet*, Vermilion, London 2014.

Wansink, Brian, *Mindless Eating: Why we eat more than we think*, Bantam, New York, 2006.

Websites

Benjamin I. Brown, ND. www.timeforwellness.org

Monash University low FODMAP diet information: www.med.monash.edu/cecs/gastro/fodmap/

Viridian Nutrition, an award-winning range of nutritional supplements available from specialist health stores: www.viridian-nutrition.com

Specialist diagnostic laboratories

Genova Diagnostics: www.gdx.net

Healthscope International Pathology, Australia: www.healthscopeinternationalpathology.com.au/

Regenerus Laboratories: www.regeneruslabs.com

REFERENCES

The digestive illness epidemic

1. Silk DB. Impact of irritable bowel syndrome on personal relationships and working practices. *Eur J Gastroenterol Hepatol.* 2001;13:1327–32.

2. Drossman DA, Morris CB, Schneck S, Hu YJ, Norton NJ, Norton WF, Weinland SR, Dalton C, Leserman J, Bangdiwala SI. International survey of patients with IBS: symptom features and their severity, health status, treatments, and risk taking to achieve clinical benefit. *J Clin Gastroenterol.* 2009 Jul;43(6):541–50.

3. Spiller RC. Irritable bowel syndrome: gender, infection, lifestyle or what else? *Dig Dis.* 2011;29(2):215–21.

4. Gwee KA, Lu CL, Ghoshal UC. Epidemiology of irritable bowel syndrome in Asia: something old, something new, something borrowed. *J Gastroenterol Hepatol.* 2009 Oct;24(10):1601–7.

5. Porter C, Cash B, Pimentel M, et al. Risk of inflammatory bowel disease following a diagnosis of irritable bowel syndrome. *BMC Gastroenterology.* 2012;12:55.

6. Guo Y, Niu K, Momma H, et al. Irritable bowel syndrome is positively related to metabolic syndrome: a population-based cross-sectional study. *PLoS One.* 2014 Nov 10;9(11):e112289.

Do you have IBS?

1. Cremonini F, Talley NJ. Irritable bowel syndrome: epidemiology, natural history, health care seeking and emerging risk factors. *Gastroenterol Clin North Am.* 2005;34(2): 189–204.

2. Talley NJ. Commentary: Controversies in NICE guidance on irritable bowel syndrome. *BMJ.* 2008 Mar 8;336(7643):558–9.

3. American College of Gastroenterology Task Force on Irritable Bowel Syndrome, Brandt LJ, Chey WD, et al. An evidence-based position statement on the management of irritable bowel syndrome. *Am J Gastroenterol.* 2009;104:S1–S35.

4. Stewart WF, Liberman JN, Sandler RS, Woods MS, Stemhagen A, Chee E, Lipton RB, Farup CE. Epidemiology of constipation (EPOC) study in the United States: relation of clinical subtypes to sociodemographic features. *Am J Gastroenterol.* 1999 Dec;94(12):3530–40.

5. Foxx-Orenstein AE, McNally MA, Odunsi ST. Update on constipation: one treatment does not fit all. *Cleve Clin J Med.* 2008 Nov;75(11):813–24.

6. Pare P, Ferrazzi S, Thompson WG, Irvine EJ, Rance L. An epidemiological survey of constipation in Canada: definitions, rates, demographics, and predictors of health care seeking. *Am J Gastroenterol.* 2001;96: 3130–7.

7. Leung L, Riutta T, Kotecha J, Rosser W. Chronic constipation: an evidence-based review. *J Am Board Fam Med.* 2011 Jul–Aug;24(4):436–51.

8. Lewis SJ, Heaton KW. Stool form scale as a useful guide to intestinal transit time. *Scand J Gastoenterol.* 1997;32: 920–4.

9. Rao SS, Kuo B, McCallum RW, Chey WD, DiBaise JK, Hasler WL, Koch KL, Lackner JM, Miller C, Saad R, Semler JR, Sitrin MD, Wilding GE, Parkman HP. Investigation of colonic and whole-gut transit with wireless motility capsule and radiopaque markers in constipation. *Clin Gastroenterol Hepatol.* 2009 May;7(5):537–44.

10. Heaton KW, O'Donnell LJ. An office guide to whole-gut transit time. Patients' recollection of their stool form. *J Clin Gastroenterol.* 1994 Jul;19(1):28–30.

11. Saad RJ, Rao SS, Koch KL, Kuo B, Parkman HP, McCallum RW, Sitrin MD, Wilding GE, Semler JR, Chey WD. Do stool form and frequency correlate with whole-gut and colonic transit? Results from a multicenter study in constipated individuals and healthy controls. *Am J Gastroenterol*. 2010 Feb;105(2):403–11.

12. Sandler RS, Stewart WF, Liberman JN, Ricci JA, Zorich NL. Abdominal pain, bloating, and diarrhea in the United States: prevalence and impact. *Dig Dis Sci*. 2000 Jun;45(6):1166–71.

13. Spiller R, Aziz Q, Creed F, Emmanuel A, Houghton L, Hungin P, Jones R, Kumar D, Rubin G, Trudgill N, Whorwell P; Clinical Services Committee of The British Society of Gastroenterology. Guidelines on the irritable bowel syndrome: mechanisms and practical management. *Gut*. 2007 Dec;56(12):1770–98.

14. Miller V, Hopkins L, Whorwell PJ. Suicidal ideation in patients with irritable bowel syndrome. *Clin Gastroenterol Hepatol*. 2004 Dec;2(12):1064–8.

15. Gorard DA, Gomborone JE, Libby GW, Farthing MJ. Intestinal transit in anxiety and depression. *Gut*. 1996 Oct;39(4):551–5.

16. Baldi F, Bianco MA, Nardone G, Pilotto A, Zamparo E. Focus on acute diarrhoeal disease. *World J Gastroenterol*. 2009 Jul 21;15(27):3341–8.

17. Chey WY, Jin HO, Lee MH, Sun SW, Lee KY. Colonic motility abnormality in patients with irritable bowel syndrome exhibiting abdominal pain and diarrhea. *Am J Gastroenterol*. 2001 May;96(5):1499–506.

18. Dunlop SP, Jenkins D, Spiller RC. Distinctive clinical, psychological, and histological features of postinfective irritable bowel syndrome. *Am J Gastroenterol*. 2003 Jul;98(7):1578–83.

19. Lembo T, Naliboff B, Munakata J, Fullerton S, Saba L, Tung S, Schmulson M, Mayer EA. Symptoms and visceral perception in patients with pain-predominant irritable bowel syndrome. *Am J Gastroenterol*. 1999 May;94(5):1320–6.

20. Agrawal A, Whorwell PJ. Review article: abdominal bloating and distention in functional gastrointestinal disorders — epidemiology and exploration of possible mechanisms. *Aliment Pharmacol Ther*. 2008 Jan 1;27(1):2–10.

21. Houghton LA, Lea R, Agrawal A, Reilly B, Whorwell PJ. Relationship of abdominal bloating to distention in irritable bowel syndrome and effect of bowel habit. *Gastroenterology.* 2006 Oct;131(4):1003–10.

22. King TS, Elia M, Hunter JO. Abnormal colonic fermentation in irritable bowel syndrome. *Lancet.* 1998; 352:1187–9.

23. Serra J, Azpiroz F, Malagelada JR. Impaired transit and tolerance of intestinal gas in the irritable bowel syndrome. *Gut.* 2001 Jan;48(1): 14–9.

24. Agrawal A, Lea R, Whorwell PJ, Houghton LA. Is visceral hyposensitivity associated with abdominal distention in Irritable Bowel Syndrome. *Gut.* 2007;56(Suppl. 2); A62,

25. Hungin AP, Whorwell PJ, Tack J, Mearin F. The prevalence, patterns and impact of irritable bowel syndrome: an international survey of 40,000 subjects. *Aliment Pharmacol Ther.* 2003;17: 643–50.

26. Creed F, Ratcliffe J, Fernandez L, Tomenson B, Palmer S, Rigby C, Guthrie E, Read N, Thompson D. Health-related quality of life and health care costs in severe, refractory irritable bowel syndrome. *Ann Intern Med.* 2001 May 1;134(9 Pt 2):860–8.

27. Katiraei P, Bultron G. Need for a comprehensive medical approach to the neuro-immuno-gastroenterology of irritable bowel syndrome. *World J Gastroenterol.* 2011 Jun 21;17(23):2791–800.

28. Mayer EA. Clinical practice. Irritable bowel syndrome. *N Engl J Med.* 2008 Apr 17;358(16):1692–9.

29. Ragnarsson G, Bodemar G. Pain is temporally related to eating but not to defaecation in the irritable bowel syndrome (IBS). Patients' description of diarrhea, constipation and symptom variation during a prospective 6-week study. *Eur J Gastroenterol Hepatol.* 1998;10(5):415–21.

30. Price DD, Craggs JG, Zhou Q, Verne GN, Perlstein WM, Robinson ME. Widespread hyperalgesia in irritable bowel syndrome is dynamically maintained by tonic visceral impulse input and placebo/ nocebo factors: evidence from human psychophysics, animal models, and neuroimaging. *Neuroimage.* 2009 Sep;47(3):995–1001.

31. Staud R, Rodriguez ME. Mechanisms of disease: pain in fibromyalgia syndrome. *Nat Clin Pract Rheumatol.* 2006 Feb;2(2):90–8.

32. Naliboff BD, Munakata J, Fullerton S, Gracely RH, Kodner A, Harraf F, Mayer EA. Evidence for two distinct perceptual alterations in irritable bowel syndrome. *Gut.* 1997 Oct;41(4):505–12.

33. Price DD, Zhou Q, Moshiree B, Robinson ME, Verne GN. Peripheral and central contributions to hyperalgesia in irritable bowel syndrome. *J Pain*. 2006 Aug;7(8):529–35.

34. Sperber AD, Atzmon Y, Neumann L, Weisberg I, Shalit Y, Abu-Shakrah M, Fich A, Buskila D. Fibromyalgia in the irritable bowel syndrome: studies of prevalence and clinical implications. *Am J Gastroenterol*. 1999 Dec;94(12):3541–6.

35. Sparkes V, Prevost AT, Hunter JO. Derivation and identification of questions that act as predictors of abdominal pain of musculoskeletal origin. *Eur J Gastroenterol Hepatol*. 2003 Sep;15(9):1021–7.

36. Henry JL. The need for knowledge translation in chronic pain. *Pain Res Manag*. 2008 Nov–Dec;13(6):465–76.

37. Julius D, Basbaum AI. Molecular mechanisms of nociception. *Nature*. 2001 Sep 13;413(6852):203–10.

38. Whorwell PJ, McCallum M, Creed FH, Roberts CT. Non-colonic features of irritable bowel syndrome. *Gut*. 1986 Jan;27(1):37–40.

39. Triadafilopoulos G, Simms RW, Goldenberg DL. Bowel dysfunction in fibromyalgia syndrome. *Dig Dis Sci*. 1991;36:59–64.

40. Sivri A, Cindas A, Dincer F, Sivri B. Bowel dysfunction and irritable bowel syndrome in fibromyalgia patients. *Clin Rheumatol*. 1996;15(3):283–6.

41. Sperber AD, Atzmon Y, Neumann L, et al. Fibromyalgia in the irritable bowel syndrome: studies of prevalence and clinical implications. *Am J Gastroenterol*. 1999;94:3541–6.

42. Sperber AD, Dekel R. Irritable Bowel Syndrome and Co-morbid Gastrointestinal and Extra-gastrointestinal Functional Syndromes. *J Neurogastroenterol Motil*. 2010 Apr;16(2):113–9.

43. Aaron LA, Burke MM, Buchwald D. Overlapping conditions among patients with chronic fatigue syndrome, fibromyalgia, and temporomandibular disorder. *Arch Intern Med*. 2000 Jan 24;160(2):221–7.

44. Gwee KA, Chua AS. Functional dyspepsia and irritable bowel syndrome, are they different entities and does it matter? *World J Gastroenterol*. 2006 May 7;12(17):2708–12.

45. Creed F, Ratcliffe J, Fernandes L, Palmer S, Rigby C, Tomenson B, Guthrie E, Read N, Thompson DG; North of England IBS Research Group. Outcome in severe irritable bowel syndrome with and without accompanying depressive, panic and neurasthenic disorders. *Br J Psychiatry*. 2005 Jun;186:507–15.

46. Lee S, Wu J, Ma YL, Tsang A, Guo WJ, Sung J. Irritable bowel syndrome is strongly associated with generalized anxiety disorder: a community study. *Aliment Pharmacol Ther*. 2009 Sep 15;30(6):643–51.

47. Mikocka-Walus AA, Turnbull DA, Andrews JM, Moulding NT, Wilson IG, Harley HA, Hetzel DJ, Holtmann GJ. Psychological problems in gastroenterology outpatients: A South Australian experience. Psychological co-morbidity in IBD, IBS and hepatitis C. *Clin Pract Epidemiol Ment Health*. 2008 May 23;4:15.

48. Surdea-Blaga T, Băban A, Dumitrascu DL. Psychosocial determinants of irritable bowel syndrome. *World J Gastroenterol*. 2012 Feb 21;18(7):616 26.

49. Goehler LE, Lyte M, Gaykema RP. Infection-induced viscerosensory signals from the gut enhance anxiety: implications for psychoneuroimmunology. *Brain Behav Immun*. 2007 Aug;21(6):721–6.

50. Fass R, Fullerton S, Naliboff B, Hirsh T, Mayer EA. Sexual dysfunction in patients with irritable bowel syndrome and non-ulcer dyspepsia. *Digestion*. 1998;59(1):79–85.

51. Longstreth GF, Yao JF. Irritable bowel syndrome and surgery: a multivariable analysis. *Gastroenterology*. 2004 Jun;126(7):1665–73.

52. Longstreth GF. Avoiding unnecessary surgery in irritable bowel syndrome. *Gut*. 2007 May;56(5):608–10.

53. Mayer EA. Clinical practice. Irritable bowel syndrome. *N Engl J Med*. 2008 Apr 17;358(16):1692–9.

54. Dalrymple J, Bullock I. Diagnosis and management of irritable bowel syndrome in adults in primary care: summary of NICE guidance. *BMJ*. 2008 Mar 8;336(7643):556–8.

55. Whitehead WE, Palsson OS, Feld AD, Levy RL, VON Korff M, Turner MJ, Drossman DA. Utility of red flag symptom exclusions in the diagnosis of irritable bowel syndrome. *Aliment Pharmacol Ther*. 2006 Jul 1;24(1):137–46.

56. Walsh JM, Terdiman JP. Colorectal cancer screening: scientific review. *JAMA*. 2003 Mar 12;289(10):1288–96.

What's going on in your gut?

1. Delvaux M. Role of visceral sensitivity in the pathophysiology of irritable bowel syndrome. *Gut*. 2002 Jul;51 Suppl 1:i67–71.

2. Zhou Q, Verne GN. New insights into visceral hypersensitivity — clinical implications in IBS. *Nat Rev Gastroenterol Hepatol*. 2011 Jun;8(6):349–55.

3. Woolf CJ. Central sensitization: implications for the diagnosis and treatment of pain. *Pain*. 2011 Mar;152(3 Suppl):S2–15.

4. Gwee KA, Chua AS. Functional dyspepsia and irritable bowel syndrome, are they different entities and does it matter? *World J Gastroenterol*. 2006 May 7;12(17):2708–12.

5. van der Voort IR, Osmanoglou E, Seybold M, Heymann-Mönnikes I, Tebbe J, Wiedenmann B, Klapp BF, Mönnikes H. Electrogastrography as a diagnostic tool for delayed gastric emptying in functional dyspepsia and irritable bowel syndrome. *Neurogastroenterol Motil*. 2003 Oct;15(5):467–73.

6. Welgan P, Meshkinpour H, Ma L. Role of anger in antral motor activity in irritable bowel syndrome. *Dig Dis Sci*. 2000 Feb;45(2):248–51.

7. Bäckhed F, Ley RE, Sonnenburg JL, Peterson DA, Gordon JI. Host-bacterial mutualism in the human intestine. *Science*. 2005 Mar 25;307(5717):1915–20.

8. Lin HC. Small intestinal bacterial overgrowth: a framework for understanding irritable bowel syndrome. *JAMA*. 2004 Aug 18;292(7):852–8.

9. Kassinen A, Krogius-Kurikka L, Makivuokko H, et al. The fecal microbiota of irritable bowel syndrome patients differs significantly from that of healthy subjects. *Gastroenterology*. 2007;133:24–33.

10. Bixquert Jiménez M. Treatment of irritable bowel syndrome with probiotics. An etiopathogenic approach at last? *Rev Esp Enferm Dig*. 2009 Aug;101(8):553–64.

11. Dahlqvist G, Piessevaux H. Irritable bowel syndrome: the role of the intestinal microbiota, pathogenesis and therapeutic targets. *Acta Gastroenterol Belg*. 2011 Sep;74(3):375–80.

12. Bixquert Jiménez M. Treatment of irritable bowel syndrome with probiotics. An etiopathogenic approach at last? *Rev Esp Enferm Dig.* 2009 Aug;101(8):553-64.

13. Ohman L, Isaksson S, Lindmark AC, Posserud I, Stotzer PO, Strid H, Sjövall H, Simrén M. T-cell activation in patients with irritable bowel syndrome. *Am J Gastroenterol.* 2009 May;104(5):1205-12.

14. Buhner S, Li Q, Vignali S, Barbara G, De Giorgio R, Stanghellini V, Cremon C, Zeller F, Langer R, Daniel H, Michel K, Schemann M. Activation of human enteric neurons by supernatants of colonic biopsy specimens from patients with irritable bowel syndrome. *Gastroenterology.* 2009 Oct;137(4):1425-34.

15. Khan WI, Collins SM. Gut motor function: immunological control in enteric infection and inflammation. *Clin Exp Immunol.* 2006 Mar;143(3):389-97.

16. Brint EK, MacSharry J, Fanning A, Shanahan F, Quigley EM. Differential expression of toll-like receptors in patients with irritable bowel syndrome. *Am J Gastroenterol.* 2011 Feb;106(2):329-36.

17. Arrieta MC, Bistritz L, Meddings JB. Alterations in intestinal permeability. *Gut.* 2006 Oct;55(10):1512-20.

18. Arrieta MC, Bistritz L, Meddings JB. Alterations in intestinal permeability. *Gut.* 2006 Oct;55(10):1512-20.

19. Shen L, Turner JR. Role of epithelial cells in initiation and propagation of intestinal inflammation. Eliminating the static: tight junction dynamics exposed. *Am J Physiol Gastrointest Liver Physiol.* 2006 Apr;290(4):G577-82.

20. Zhou Q, Zhang B, Verne GN. Intestinal membrane permeability and hypersensitivity in the irritable bowel syndrome. *Pain.* 2009 Nov;146(1-2):41-6.

21. Barbara G. Mucosal barrier defects in irritable bowel syndrome. Who left the door open? *Am J Gastroenterol.* 2006 Jun;101(6):1295-8.

22. Zhou Q, Zhang B, Verne GN. Intestinal membrane permeability and hypersensitivity in the irritable bowel syndrome. *Pain.* 2009 Nov;146(1-2):41-6.

23. Dunlop SP, Hebden J, Campbell E, Naesdal J, Olbe L, Perkins AC, Spiller RC. Abnormal intestinal permeability in subgroups of diarrhea-predominant irritable bowel syndromes. *Am J Gastroenterol.* 2006 Jun;101(6):1288–94. Erratum in: *Am J Gastroenterol.* 2006 Aug;101(8):1944.

24. Konturek PC, Brzozowski T, Konturek SJ. Stress and the gut: pathophysiology, clinical consequences, diagnostic approach and treatment options. *J Physiol Pharmacol.* 2011 Dec;62(6):591–9.

25. Chang L. The role of stress on physiologic responses and clinical symptoms in irritable bowel syndrome. *Gastroenterology.* 2011 Mar;140(3):761–5. Epub 2011 Jan 19.

26. Kennedy PJ, Clarke G, Quigley EM, Groeger JA, Dinan TG, Cryan JF. Gut memories: towards a cognitive neurobiology of irritable bowel syndrome. *Neurosci Biobehav Rev.* 2012 Jan;36(1):310–40. Epub 2011 Jul 13.

27. Bercik P, Park AJ, Sinclair D, Khoshdel A, Lu J, Huang X, Deng Y, Blennerhassett PA, Fahnestock M, Moine D, Berger B, Huizinga JD, Kunze W, McLean PG, Bergonzelli GE, Collins SM, Verdu EF. The anxiolytic effect of Bifidobacterium longum NCC3001 involves vagal pathways for gut-brain communication. *Neurogastroenterol Motil.* 2011 Dec;23(12):1132–9.

Banish bad bugs and balance your bacteria

1. Hawrelak JA, Myers SP. The causes of intestinal dysbiosis: a review. *Altern Med Rev.* 2004 Jun;9(2):180–97.

2. Ghoshal UC, Shukla R, Ghoshal U, Gwee KA, Ng SC, Quigley EM. The gut microbiota and irritable bowel syndrome: friend or foe? *Int J Inflam.* 2012;2012:151085.

3. Pimentel M, Chow EJ, Lin HC. Normalization of lactulose breath testing correlates with symptom improvement in irritable bowel syndrome. a double-blind, randomized, placebo-controlled study. *Am J Gastroenterol.* 2003 Feb;98(2):412–9.

4. Pimentel M, Lembo A, Chey WD, Zakko S, Ringel Y, Yu J, Mareya SM, Shaw AL, Bortey E, Forbes WP; TARGET Study Group. Rifaximin therapy for patients with irritable bowel syndrome without constipation. *N Engl J Med.* 2011 Jan 6;364(1):22–32.

5. Lin HC. Small intestinal bacterial overgrowth: a framework for understanding irritable bowel syndrome. *JAMA*. 2004 Aug 18;292(7):852–8.

6. Dukowicz AC, Lacy BE, Levine GM. Small intestinal bacterial overgrowth: a comprehensive review. *Gastroenterol Hepatol* (NY). 2007 Feb;3(2):112–22.

7. Pyleris E, Giamarellos-Bourboulis EJ, Tzivras D, Koussoulas V, Barbatzas C, Pimentel M. The prevalence of overgrowth by aerobic bacteria in the small intestine by small bowel culture: relationship with irritable bowel syndrome. *Dig Dis Sci*. 2012 May; 57(5):1321–9 Epub 2012 Jan 20.

8. Lin HC. Small intestinal bacterial overgrowth: a framework for understanding irritable bowel syndrome. *JAMA*. 2004 Aug 18;292(7):852–8.

9. Haboubi NY, Lee GS, Montgomery RD. Duodenal mucosal morphometry of elderly patients with small intestinal bacterial overgrowth: response to antibiotic treatment. *Age Ageing*. 1991 Jan;20(1):29–32.

10. Reddymasu SC, Sostarich S, McCallum RW. Small intestinal bacterial overgrowth in irritable bowel syndrome: are there any predictors? *BMC Gastroenterol*. 2010 Feb 22;10:23.

11. Collins BS, Lin HC. Chronic abdominal pain in children is associated with high prevalence of abnormal microbial fermentation. *Dig Dis Sci*. 2010 Jan;55(1):124–30.

12. Bures J, Cyrany J, Kohoutova D, Förstl M, Rejchrt S, Kvetina J, Vorisek V, Kopacova M. Small intestinal bacterial overgrowth syndrome. *World J Gastroenterol*. 2010 Jun 28;16(24):2978–90.

13. Pimentel M, Wallace D, Hallegua D, Chow E, Kong Y, Park S, Lin HC. A link between irritable bowel syndrome and fibromyalgia may be related to findings on lactulose breath testing. *Ann Rheum Dis* 2004;63:450–452.

14. Rubio-Tapia A, Barton SH, Rosenblatt JE, Murray JA. Prevalence of small intestine bacterial overgrowth diagnosed by quantitative culture of intestinal aspirate in celiac disease. *J Clin Gastroenterol* 2009;43:157–61.

15. Almeida JA, Kim R, Stoita A, McIver CJ, Kurtovic J, Riordan SM. Lactose malabsorption in the elderly: role of small intestinal bacterial overgrowth. *Scand J Gastroenterol* 2008;43:146–154.

16. Teo M, Chung S, Chitti L, Tran C, Kritas S, Butler R, Cummins A. Small bowel bacterial overgrowth is a common cause of chronic diarrhea. *J Gastroenterol Hepatol*. 2004 Aug;19(8):904–9.

17. Sachdeva S, Rawat AK, Reddy RS, Puri AS. Small intestinal bacterial overgrowth (SIBO) in irritable bowel syndrome: frequency and predictors. *J Gastroenterol Hepatol*. 2011 Apr;26 Suppl 3:135–8.

18. Lewis SJ, Franco S, Young G, O'Keefe SJ. Altered bowel function and duodenal bacterial overgrowth in patients treated with omeprazole. *Aliment Pharmacol Ther*. 1996 Aug;10(4):557–61.

19. Spiegel BM, Chey WD, Chang L. Bacterial overgrowth and irritable bowel syndrome: unifying hypothesis or a spurious consequence of proton pump inhibitors? *Am J Gastroenterol*. 2008 Dec;103(12):2972–6.

20. Compare D, Pica L, Rocco A, De Giorgi F, Cuomo R, Sarnelli G, Romano M, Nardone G. Effects of long-term PPI treatment on producing bowel symptoms and SIBO. *Eur J Clin Invest*. 2011 Apr;41(4):380–6.

21. Kelly GS. Hydrochloric acid: physiological functions and clinical implications. *Alt Med Rev*. 1997;2(2):116–127.

22. Reddymasu SC, Sostarich S, McCallum RW. Small intestinal bacterial overgrowth in irritable bowel syndrome: are there any predictors? *BMC Gastroenterol*. 2010 Feb 22;10:23.

23. Tursi A, Brandimarte G, Giorgetti G. High prevalence of small intestinal bacterial overgrowth in celiac patients with persistence of gastrointestinal symptoms after gluten withdrawal. *Am J Gastroenterol*. 2003 Apr;98(4):839–43.

24. Rubio-Tapia A, Barton SH, Rosenblatt JE, Murray JA. Prevalence of small intestine bacterial overgrowth diagnosed by quantitative culture of intestinal aspirate in celiac disease. *J Clin Gastroenterol*. 2009 Feb;43(2):157–61.

25. Quigley EM. Do patients with functional gastrointestinal disorders have an altered gut flora? *Therap Adv Gastroenterol*. 2009 Jul;2(4):23–30.

26. Quigley EM. Do patients with functional gastrointestinal disorders have an altered gut flora? *Therap Adv Gastroenterol*. 2009 Jul;2(4):23–30.

27. Jalanka-Tuovinen J, Salonen A, Nikkilä J, Immonen O, Kekkonen R, Lahti L, Palva A, de Vos WM. Intestinal microbiota in healthy adults: temporal analysis reveals individual and common core and relation to intestinal symptoms. *PLoS One*. 2011;6(7):e23035.

28. Kassinen A, Krogius-Kurikka L, Makivuokko H, et al. The fecal microbiota of irritable bowel syndrome patients differs significantly from that of healthy subjects. *Gastroenterology*. 2007;133:24–33.

29. Maukonen J, Satokari R, Mättö J, Söderlund H, Mattila-Sandholm T, Saarela M. Prevalence and temporal stability of selected clostridial groups in irritable bowel syndrome in relation to predominant faecal bacteria. *J Med Microbiol*. 2006 May;55(Pt 5):625–33.

30. Rinttilä T, Lyra A, Krogius-Kurikka L, Palva A. Real-time PCR analysis of enteric pathogens from fecal samples of irritable bowel syndrome subjects. *Gut Pathog*. 2011 Apr 26;3(1):6.

31. Shanahan F. Irritable bowel syndrome: shifting the focus toward the gut microbiota. *Gastroenterology*. 2007 Jul;133(1):340–2.

32. Niedzielin K, Kordecki H, Birkenfeld B. A controlled, double-blind, randomized study on the efficacy of Lactobacillus plantarum 299V in patients with irritable bowel syndrome. *Eur J Gastroenterol Hepatol*. 2001 Oct;13(10):1143–7.

33. Thabane M, Marshall JK. Post-infectious irritable bowel syndrome. *World J Gastroenterol*. 2009 Aug 7;15(29):3591–6.

34. Thabane M, Kottachchi DT, Marshall JK. Systematic review and meta-analysis: The incidence and prognosis of post-infectious irritable bowel syndrome. *Aliment Pharmacol Ther*. 2007 Aug 15;26(4):535–44.

35. Ghoshal UC, Shukla R, Ghoshal U, Gwee KA, Ng SC, Quigley EM. The gut microbiota and irritable bowel syndrome: friend or foe? *Int J Inflam*. 2012;2012:151085.

36. Hanevik K, Dizdar V, Langeland N, Hausken T. Development of functional gastrointestinal disorders after Giardia lamblia infection. *BMC Gastroenterol*. 2009 Apr 21;9:27.

37. Nygård K, Schimmer B, Søbstad Ø, Walde A, Tveit I, Langeland N, Hausken T, Aavitsland P. A large community outbreak of waterborne giardiasis-delayed detection in a non-endemic urban area. *BMC Public Health*. 2006 May 25;6:141.

38. Wensaas KA, Langeland N, Hanevik K, Mørch K, Eide GE, Rortveit G. Irritable bowel syndrome and chronic fatigue 3 years after acute giardiasis: historic cohort study. *Gut*. 2012 Feb;61(2):214–9.

39. Hanevik K, Dizdar V, Langeland N, Hausken T. Development of functional gastrointestinal disorders after Giardia lamblia infection. *BMC Gastroenterol*. 2009 Apr 21;9:27.

40. DuPont AW. Postinfectious irritable bowel syndrome. *Clin Infect Dis*. 2008 Feb 15;46(4):594–9.

41. Leder K, Hellard ME, Sinclair MI, et al. No correlation between clinical symptoms and *Blastocystis hominis* in immunocompetent individuals. *J Gastroenterol Hepatol*. 2005 Sep;20(9):1390–4.

42. Poirier P, Wawrzyniak I, Vivarès CP, et al. New insights into *Blastocystis spp.*: a potential link with irritable bowel syndrome. *PLoS Pathog*. 2012;8(3):e1002545.

43. Nourrisson C, Scanzi J, Pereira B, et al. *Blastocystis* is associated with decrease of fecal microbiota protective bacteria: comparative analysis between patients with irritable bowel syndrome and control subjects. *PLoS One*. 2014 Nov 3;9(11):e111868.

44. Ragavan ND, Govind SK, Chye TT, Mahadeva S. Phenotypic variation in *Blastocystis sp*. ST3. *Parasit Vectors*. 2014 Aug 29;7:404.

45. Vargas-Sanchez GB, Romero-Valdovinos M, Ramirez-Guerrero C, et al. *Blastocystis* isolates from patients with irritable bowel syndrome and from asymptomatic carriers exhibit similar parasitological loads, but significantly different generation times and genetic variability across multiple subtypes. *PLoS One*. 2015 Apr 29;10(4):e0124006.

46. Kuo HY, Chiang DH, Wang CC, et al. Clinical significance of *Blastocystis hominis*: experience from a medical center in northern Taiwan. *J Microbiol Immunol Infect*. 2008 Jun;41(3):222–6.

47. Truss CO. Tissue injury induced by Candida albicans, mental and neurological manifestations. *J Orthomol Psychiatry*. 1978;7:17–37.

48. Crook WG. *The Yeast Connection*. Jackson, TN: Professional Books; 1983.

49. Dismukes WE, Wade JS, Lee JY, Dockery BK, Hain JD. A randomized, double-blind trial of nystatin therapy for the candidiasis hypersensitivity syndrome. *N Engl J Med*. 1990 Dec 20;323(25): 1717–23.

50. Lacour M, Zunder T, Huber R, Sander A, Daschner F, Frank U. The pathogenetic significance of intestinal Candida colonization — a systematic review from an interdisciplinary and environmental medical point of view. *Int J Hyg Environ Health.* 2002 May;205(4):257–68.

51. Crook WG. A controlled trial of nystatin for the candidiasis hypersensitivity syndrome. *N Engl J Med.* 1991 May 30;324(22):1592–4.

52. Crandall M. The pathogenetic significance of intestinal Candida colonization. *Int J Hyg Environ Health.* 2004 Jan;207(1):79–81.

53. Gaby, AR. Candidiasis, in *Nutritional Medicine.* Fritz Pelberg Publishing. Concord, NH. 2011.

54. Rucklidge JJ. Could yeast infections impair recovery from mental illness? A case study using micronutrients and olive leaf extract for the treatment of ADHD and depression. *Adv Mind Body Med.* 2013 Summer;27(3):14–8.

55. Scanlan PD, Marchesi JR. Micro-eukaryotic diversity of the human distal gut microbiota: qualitative assessment using culture-dependent and -independent analysis of faeces. *ISME J.* 2008;2(12):1183–93.

56. Li Q, Wang C, Tang C, He Q, Li N, Li J. Dysbiosis of gut fungal microbiota is associated with mucosal inflammation in Crohn's disease. *J Clin Gastroenterol.* 2014 Jul;48(6):513–23.

57. Kumamoto CA. Inflammation and gastrointestinal Candida colonization. *Curr Opin Microbiol.* 2011 Aug;14(4):386–91.

58. Mendall MA, Kumar D. Antibiotic use, childhood affluence and irritable bowel syndrome (IBS). *Eur J Gastroenterol Hepatol.* 1998;10:59–62.

59. Gaby, AR. Candidiasis, in *Nutritional Medicine.* Fritz Pelberg Publishing. Concord, NH. 2011

60. Santelmann H, Laerum E, Roennevig J, Fagertun HE. Effectiveness of nystatin in polysymptomatic patients: a randomized, double-blind trial with nystatin versus placebo in general practice. *Fam Pract.* 2001 Jun;18(3):258–65.

61. Ligaarden SC, Axelsson L, Naterstad K, Lydersen S, Farup PG. A candidate probiotic with unfavourable effects in subjects with irritable bowel syndrome: a randomised controlled trial. *BMC Gastroenterol.* 2010 Feb 10;10:16.

62. Niv E, Naftali T, Hallak R, Vaisman N. The efficacy of Lactobacillus reuteri ATCC 55730 in the treatment of patients with irritable bowel syndrome — a double blind, placebo-controlled, randomized study. *Clin Nutr.* 2005 Dec;24(6):925–31.

63. Bausserman M, Michail S. The use of Lactobacillus GG in irritable bowel syndrome in children: a double-blind randomized control trial. *J Pediatr.* 2005 Aug;147(2):197–201.

64. McFarland LV, Dublin S. Meta-analysis of probiotics for the treatment of irritable bowel syndrome. *World J Gastroenterol.* 2008 May 7;14(17):2650–61.

65. Haller D, et al. Guidance for substantiating the evidence for beneficial effects of probiotics: probiotics in chronic inflammatory bowel disease and the functional disorder irritable bowel syndrome. *J Nutr.* 2010 Mar;140(3):690S–7S.

66. Stotzer PO, Blomberg L, Conway PL, Henriksson A, Abrahamsson H. Probiotic treatment of small intestinal bacterial overgrowth by Lactobacillus fermentum KLD. *Scand J Infect Dis.* 1996;28(6):615–9.

67. Barrett JS, Canale KE, Gearry RB, Irving PM, Gibson PR. Probiotic effects on intestinal fermentation patterns in patients with irritable bowel syndrome. *World J Gastroenterol.* 2008 Aug 28;14(32):5020–4.

68. Gabrielli M, Lauritano EC, Scarpellini E, Lupascu A, Ojetti V, Gasbarrini G, Silveri NG, Gasbarrini A. Bacillus clausii as a treatment of small intestinal bacterial overgrowth. *Am J Gastroenterol.* 2009 May;104(5):1327–8.

69. Schiffrin EJ, Parlesak A, Bode C, Bode JC, van't Hof MA, Grathwohl D, Guigoz Y. Probiotic yogurt in the elderly with intestinal bacterial overgrowth: endotoxaemia and innate immune functions. *Br J Nutr.* 2009 Apr;101(7):961–6.

70. Soifer LO, Peralta D, Dima G, Besasso H. Comparative clinical efficacy of a probiotic vs. an antibiotic in the treatment of patients with intestinal bacterial overgrowth and chronic abdominal functional distention: a pilot study. *Acta Gastroenterol Latinoam.* 2010 Dec;40(4):323–7.

71. Roberfroid M, Gibson GR, Hoyles L, et al. Prebiotic effects: metabolic and health benefits. *Br J Nutr.* 2010 Aug;104 Suppl 2:S1–63.

72. Poutanen K, Flander L, Katina K. Sourdough and cereal fermentation in a nutritional perspective. *Food Microbiol.* 2009 Oct;26(7):693–9.

73. Costabile A, Santarelli S, Claus SP, et al. Effect of breadmaking process on in vitro gut microbiota parameters in irritable bowel syndrome. *PLoS One.* 2014 Oct 30;9(10):e111225.

74. Sõukand R, Pieroni A, Biró M, et al. An ethnobotanical perspective on traditional fermented plant foods and beverages in Eastern Europe. *J Ethnopharmacol.* 2015 Jul 21;170:284–96.

75. Leroy F, De Vuyst L. Fermented food in the context of a healthy diet: how to produce novel functional foods? *Curr Opin Clin Nutr Metab Care.* 2014 Nov;17(6):574–81.

76. Han K, Bose S, Wang JH, et al. Contrasting effects of fresh and fermented kimchi consumption on gut microbiota composition and gene expression related to metabolic syndrome in obese Korean women. *Mol Nutr Food Res.* 2015 May;59(5):1004–8.

77. Zheng Y, Lu Y, Wang J, et al. Probiotic properties of *Lactobacillus* strains isolated from Tibetan kefir grains. *PLoS One.* 2013 Jul 22;8(7):e69868.

78. Ostadrahimi A, Taghizadeh A, Mobasseri M, et al. Effect of probiotic fermented milk (kefir) on glycemic control and lipid profile in type 2 diabetic patients: a randomized double-blind placebo-controlled clinical trial. *Iran J Public Health.* 2015 Feb;44(2):228–37.

79. Kim EK, An SY, Lee MS, et al. Fermented kimchi reduces body weight and improves metabolic parameters in overweight and obese patients. *Nutr Res.* 2011 Jun;31(6):436–43.

80. Hertzler SR, Clancy SM. Kefir improves lactose digestion and tolerance in adults with lactose maldigestion. *J Am Diet Assoc.* 2003; 103: 582–7.

81. Bakken JS. Staggered and tapered antibiotic withdrawal with administration of kefir for recurrent Clostridium difficile infection. *Clin Infect Dis.* 2014 Sep 15;59(6):858–61.

82. Turan İ, Dedeli Ö, Bor S, İlter T. Effects of a kefir supplement on symptoms, colonic transit, and bowel satisfaction score in patients with chronic constipation: a pilot study. *Turk J Gastroenterol.* 2014 Dec;25(6):650–6.

83. Shen YH, Nahas R. Complementary and alternative medicine for treatment of irritable bowel syndrome. *Can Fam Physician.* 2009 Feb;55(2):143–8.

84. Logan AC, Beaulne TM. The treatment of small intestinal bacterial overgrowth with enteric-coated peppermint oil: a case report. *Altern Med Rev*. 2002 Oct; 7(5):410–7.

85. Chedid V, Dhalla S, Clarke JO, et al. Herbal therapy is equivalent to rifaximin for the treatment of small intestinal bacterial overgrowth. *Glob Adv Health Med*. 2014 May;3(3):16–24

86. Stensvold CR, Smith HV, Nagel R, et al. Eradication of *Blastocystis* carriage with antimicrobials: reality or delusion? *J Clin Gastroenterol*. 2010 Feb;44(2):85–90.

87. Borody TJ, Warren EF, Wettstein A, et al. Eradication of *Dientamoeba fragilis* can resolve IBS-like symptoms. *J Gastroenterol Hepatol*.2002;17:A103.

88. Nigro L, Larocca L, Massarelli L, et al. A placebo controlled treatment trial of *Blastocystis hominis* infection with metronidazole. *J Travel Med*. 2003;10:128–30.

89. Dinleyici EC, Eren M, Dogan N, et al. Clinical efficacy of *Saccharomyces boulardii* or metronidazole in symptomatic children with *Blastocystis hominis* infection. *Parasitol Res*. 2011 nMar;108(3):541–5.

90. El Wakil SS. Evaluation of the in vitro effect of Nigella sativa aqueous extract on *Blastocystis hominis* isolates. *J Egypt Soc Parasitol*. 2007 Dec;37(3):801–13.

91. Yang LQ, Singh M, Yap EH, et al. In vitro response of *Blastocystis hominis* against traditional Chinese medicine. *J Ethnopharmacol*. 1996 Dec;55(1):35–42.

92. Chen C, Tao C, Liu Y, et al. A randomized clinical trial of berberine hydrochloride in patients with diarrhea-predominant irritable bowel syndrome. *Phytother Res*. 2015 Sep 24. doi: 10.1002/ptr.5475.

93. Force M, Sparks WS, Ronzio RA. Inhibition of enteric parasites by emulsified oil of oregano in vivo. *Phytother Res*. 2000 May;14(3): 213–4.

94. Salem EM, Yar T, Bamosa AO, et al. Comparative study of *Nigella sativa* and triple therapy in eradication of *Helicobacter pylori* in patients with non-ulcer dyspepsia. *Saudi J Gastroenterol*. 2010 Jul-Sep;16(3):207–14.

95. Gaby, AR. Candidiasis, in *Nutritional Medicine*. Fritz Pelberg Publishing. Concord, NH. 2011.

96. Bruni N, Capucchio MT, Biasibetti E, et al. Antimicrobial activity of lactoferrin-related peptides and applications in human and veterinary medicine. *Molecules*. 2016 Jun 11;21(6).

97. Quigley EM, Abu-Shanab A. Small intestinal bacterial overgrowth. *Infect Dis Clin North Am*. 2010 Dec;24(4):943–59, viii–ix.

98. Menees SB, Maneerattannaporn M, Kim HM, Chey WD. The efficacy and safety of rifaximin for the irritable bowel syndrome: a systematic review and meta-analysis. *Am J Gastroenterol*. 2012 Jan;107(1):28–35.

99. Cremonini F, Lembo A. Rifaximin for the treatment of irritable bowel syndrome. *Expert Opin Pharmacother*. 2012 Feb;13(3):433–40.

100. Farrell DJ. Rifaximin in the treatment of irritable bowel syndrome: is there a high risk for development of antimicrobial resistance? *J Clin Gastroenterol*. 2013 Mar;47(3):205–11.

Boost your digestion for better health

1. Gaby, AR. Hypochlorhydria, in *Nutritional Medicine*. Fritz Pelberg Publishing. Concord, NH. 2011.

2. Sharp GS, Fister HW. The diagnosis and treatment of achlorhydria: ten-year study. *J Amer Ger Soc* 1967;15:786–791.

3. Brummer P, Kasanen A. The effect of hydrochloric acid on the indican metabolism in achlorhydria. *Acta Med Scand*. 1956 Jun 30;155(1):11–4.

4. Pounder RE, Fraser AG. Gastric acid secretion and intragastric acidity: measurement in health and disease. *Baillieres Clin Gastroenterol*. 1993 Mar;7(1):55–80.

5. Gerards C, Leodolter A, Glasbrenner B, Malfertheiner P. H. pylori infection and visceral hypersensitivity in patients with irritable bowel syndrome. *Dig Dis*. 2001;19(2):170–3.

6. Compare D, Pica L, Rocco A, De Giorgi F, Cuomo R, Sarnelli G, Romano M, Nardone G. Effects of long-term PPI treatment on producing bowel symptoms and SIBO. *Eur J Clin Invest*. 2011 Apr;41(4):380–6.

7. Leeds JS, Hopper AD, Sidhu R, Simmonette A, Azadbakht N, Hoggard N, Morley S, Sanders DS. Some patients with irritable bowel syndrome may have exocrine pancreatic insufficiency. *Clin Gastroenterol Hepatol*. 2010 May;8(5):433–8.

8. Money ME, Walkowiak J, Virgilio C, Talley NJ. Pilot study: a randomised, double blind, placebo controlled trial of pancrealipase for the treatment of postprandial irritable bowel syndrome-diarrhoea. *Frontline Gastroenterol.* 2011 Jan;2(1):48–56.

9. Suarez F, Levitt MD, Adshead J, Barkin JS. Pancreatic supplements reduce symptomatic response of healthy subjects to a high fat meal. *Dig Dis Sci.* 1999 Jul;44(7):1317–21.

10. Money ME, Hofmann AF, Hagey LR, Walkowiak J, Talley NJ. Treatment of irritable bowel syndrome-diarrhea with pancrealipase or colesevelam and association with steatorrhea. *Pancreas.* 2009 Mar;38(2):232–3.

11. Braganza JM, Lee SH, McCloy RF, McMahon MJ. Chronic pancreatitis. *Lancet.* 2011 Apr 2;377(9772):1184–97.

12. Walters JR, Pattni SS. Managing bile acid diarrhoea. *Therap Adv Gastroenterol.* 2010 Nov;3(6):349–57.

13. Wedlake L, A'Hern R, Russell D, Thomas K, Walters JR, Andreyev HJ. Systematic review: the prevalence of idiopathic bile acid malabsorption as diagnosed by SeHCAT scanning in patients with diarrhoea-predominant irritable bowel syndrome. *Aliment Pharmacol Ther.* 2009 Oct;30(7):707–17.

14. Walters JR, Pattni SS. Managing bile acid diarrhoea. *Therap Adv Gastroenterol.* 2010 Nov;3(6):349–57.

15. Roberts SH, James O, Jarvis EH. Bacterial overgrowth syndrome without 'blind loop': A cause for malnutrition in the elderly. *Lancet.* 1977 Dec 10;2(8050):1193–5.

16. Prousky JE. Cobalamin deficiency in elderly patients. *CMAJ.* 2005 Feb 15;172(4):450–1.

17. Yago MA, Frymoyer A, Smelick GS, Frassetto LA, Budha N, Dresser MJ, Ware J, Benet LZ. Gastric re-acidification with betaine HCl in healthy volunteers with rabeprazole-induced hypochlorhydria. *Mol Pharm.* 2013 Aug 27. [Epub ahead of print]

18. Gebhardt, R. Stimulation of acid secretion by extracts of *Gentiana lutea L.* in cultured cells from rat gastric mucosa. *Pharmaceutical and Pharmacological Letters.* 1997 7(2–3): 106–108.

19. Bradley PR, ed. *British Herbal Compendium: A handbook of scientific information on widely used plant drugs.* (vol. 1) Guilford and King's Lynn, Great Britain: Biddles Ltd; 1992:109–111.

20. Knöss, W.,Stolte, F. 2009b. Community herbal monographon *Gentian lutea L.*, radix. European Medicines Agency, London.

21. Roxas M. The role of enzyme supplementation in digestive disorders. *Altern Med Rev.* 2008;13(4):307–14.

22. Resnick C (2012). Microbial Enzyme Therapy. In JE Pizzorno and MT Murray (Eds.), *Textbook of Natural Medicine* 4 edn. (pp.876–881). Churchill Livingstone.

23. Money ME, Camilleri M. Review: management of postprandial diarrhea syndrome. *Am J Med.* 2012 Jun;125(6):538–44.

24. Westergaard H. Bile acid malabsorption. *Curr Treat Options Gastroenterol.* 2007 Feb;10(1):28–33.

25. Stenman LK, Holma R, Korpela R. High-fat-induced intestinal permeability dysfunction associated with altered fecal bile acids. *World J Gastroenterol.* 2012 Mar 7;18(9):923–9.

26. Cummings JH, Wiggins HS, Jenkins DJ, Houston H, Jivraj T, Drasar BS, Hill MJ. Influence of diets high and low in animal fat on bowel habit, gastrointestinal transit time, fecal microflora, bile acid, and fat excretion. *J Clin Invest.* 1978 Apr;61(4):953–63.

27. Fried M, Jansen JB, Harpole T, et al. Pancreatobiliary responses to an intragastric amino acid meal: comparison to albumin, dextrose, and a maximal cholecystokinin stimulus. *Gastroenterology.* 1989;97:1544–9.

28. Gråsten SM, Juntunen KS, Poutanen KS, Gylling HK, Miettinen TA, Mykkänen HM. Rye bread improves bowel function and decreases the concentrations of some compounds that are putative colon cancer risk markers in middle-aged women and men. *J Nutr.* 2000 Sep;130(9):2215–21.

29. Nagengast FM, van den Ban G, Ploemen JP, Leenen R, Zock PL, Katan MB, Hectors MP, de Haan AF, van Tongeren JH. The effect of a natural high-fibre diet on faecal and biliary bile acids, faecal pH and whole-gut transit time in man. A controlled study. *Eur J Clin Nutr.* 1993 Sep;47(9):631–9.

30. Spiller GA, Story JA, Lodics TA, Pollack M, Monyan S, Butterfield G, Spiller M. Effect of sun-dried raisins on bile acid excretion, intestinal transit time, and fecal weight: a dose-response study. *J Med Food.* 2003 Summer;6(2):87–91.

Clear constipation and reboot your system

1. Bassotti G, Carlani E, Baldón M, Gullà N, Morozzi B, Villanacci V. Painful constipation: a neglected entity? *Rev Esp Enferm Dig.* 2011 Jan;103(1):25–8.

2. Hunter JO. *Irritable bowel solutions: the essential guide to irritable bowel syndrome, its causes and treatments.* Vermilion, London, 2007.

3. Raahave D, Loud FB. Additional faecal reservoirs or hidden constipation: a link between functional and organic bowel disease. *Dan Med Bull.* 2004 Nov;51(4):422–5.

4. Raahave D, Christensen E, Loud FB, Knudsen LL. Correlation of bowel symptoms with colonic transit, length, and faecal load in functional faecal retention. *Dan Med Bull.* 2009 May;56(2):83–8.

5. Nurko S, Scott SM. Coexistence of constipation and incontinence in children and adults. *Best Pract Res Clin Gastroenterol.* 2011 Feb;25(1):29–41.

6. Foxx-Orenstein AE, McNally MA, Odunsi ST. Update on constipation: one treatment does not fit all. *Cleve Clin J Med.* 2008 Nov;75(11):813–24.

7. Chmielewska A, Szajewska H. Systematic review of randomised controlled trials: probiotics for functional constipation. *World J Gastroenterol.* 2010 Jan 7;16(1):69–75.

8. Oztürk R, Rao SS. Defecation disorders: an important subgroup of functional constipation, its pathophysiology, evaluation and treatment with biofeedback. *Turk J Gastroenterol.* 2007 Sep;18(3):139–49.

9. Mulak A, Paradowski L. Anorectal function and dyssynergic defecation in different subgroups of patients with irritable bowel syndrome. *Int J Colorectal Dis.* 2010 Aug;25(8):1011–6.

10. Lembo A, Camilleri M. Chronic constipation. *N Engl J Med.* 2003 Oct 2;349(14):1360–8.

11. Spiller R, Aziz Q, Creed F, Emmanuel A, Houghton L, Hungin P, Jones R, Kumar D, Rubin G, Trudgill N, Whorwell P; Clinical Services Committee of The British Society of Gastroenterology. Guidelines on the irritable bowel syndrome: mechanisms and practical management. *Gut.* 2007 Dec;56(12):1770–98.

12. Kearney DJ, Brown-Chang J. Complementary and alternative medicine for IBS in adults: mind-body interventions. *Nat Clin Pract Gastroenterol Hepatol*. 2008 Nov;5(11):624–36.

13. Carroccio A, Di Prima L, Iacono G, Florena AM, D'Arpa F, Sciumè C, Cefalù AB, Noto D, Averna MR. Multiple food hypersensitivity as a cause of refractory chronic constipation in adults. *Scand J Gastroenterol*. 2006 Apr;41(4):498–504.

14. Carroccio A, Iacono G. Review article: Chronic constipation and food hypersensitivity — an intriguing relationship. *Aliment Pharmacol Ther*. 2006 Nov 1;24(9):1295–304.

15. Rush EC, Patel M, Plank LD, Ferguson LR. Kiwifruit promotes laxation in the elderly. *Asia Pac J Clin Nutr*. 2002;11(2):164–8.

16. Chan AO, Leung G, Tong T, Wong NY. Increasing dietary fiber intake in terms of kiwifruit improves constipation in Chinese patients. *World J Gastroenterol*. 2007 Sep 21;13(35):4771–5.

17. Chang CC, Lin YT, Lu YT, Liu YS, Liu JF. Kiwifruit improves bowel function in patients with irritable bowel syndrome with constipation. *Asia Pac J Clin Nutr*. 2010;19(4):451–7.

18. Udani JK, Bloom DW. Effects of Kivia powder on gut health in patients with occasional constipation: a randomized, double-blind, placebo-controlled study. *Nutr J*. 2013 Jun 8;12:78.

19. Drummond L, Gearry RB. Kiwifruit modulation of gastrointestinal motility. *Adv Food Nutr Res*. 2013;68:219–32.

20. Moughan PJ, Rutherfurd SM, Balan P. Kiwifruit, mucins, and the gut barrier. *Adv Food Nutr Res*. 2013;68:169–85.

21. Kaur L, Boland M. Influence of kiwifruit on protein digestion. *Adv Food Nutr Res*. 2013;68:149–67.

22. Muss C, Mosgoeller W, Endler T. Papaya preparation (Caricol®) in digestive disorders. *Neuro Endocrinol Lett*. 2013;34(1):38–46.

23. Cockerell KM, Watkins ASM, Reeves LB, Goddard L & Lomer MCE. Effects of linseeds on the symptoms of irritable bowel syndrome: a pilot randomised controlled trial. *J Hum Nutr Diet*. 2012;25:435–443.

24. Tarpila, S, Tarpila, A, Grohn, P, Silvennoinen, T & Lindberg, L. Efficacy of ground flaxseed on constipation in patients with irritable bowel syndrome. *Curr Top Nutraceut*. 2004; Res. 2:119–125.

25. Choi CH, Chang SK. Alteration of gut microbiota and efficacy of probiotics in functional constipation. *J Neurogastroenterol Motil.* 2015 Jan 31;21(1):4–7.

26. Dimidi E, Christodoulides S, Fragkos KC, et al. The effect of probiotics on functional constipation in adults: a systematic review and meta-analysis of randomized controlled trials. *Am J Clin Nutr.* 2014 Oct;100(4):107–84.

27. Waller PA, Gopal PK, Leyer GJ, et al. Dose-response effect of Bifidobacterium lactis HN019 on whole gut transit time and functional gastrointestinal symptoms in adults. *Scand J Gastroenterol.* 2011 Sep;46(9):1057–64.

28. Kim SE, Choi SC, Park KS, et al. Change of fecal flora and effectiveness of the short-term VSL#3 probiotic treatment in patients with functional constipation. *J Neurogastroenterol Motil.* 2015 Jan 1;21(1):111–20.

29. Ojetti V, Ianiro G, Tortora A, et al. The effect of Lactobacillus reuteri supplementation in adults with chronic functional constipation: a randomized, double-blind, placebo-controlled trial. *J Gastrointestin Liver Dis.* 2014 Dec;23(4):387–91.

30. Ford AC, Quigley EM, Lacy BE, et al. Efficacy of prebiotics, probiotics, and synbiotics in irritable bowel syndrome and chronic idiopathic constipation: systematic review and meta-analysis. *Am J Gastroenterol.* 2014 Oct;109(10):1547–61.

31. Pasalar M, Lankarani KB. Letter: prunes for the treatment of constipation. *Aliment Pharmacol Ther.* 2015 Jan;41(2):234.

32. Attaluri A, et al. Dried plums, constipation and the irritable bowel syndrome: authors' reply. *Aliment Pharmacol Ther* 2011; 34: 397–8.

33. Attaluri A, Donahoe R, Valestin J, Brown K, Rao SS. Randomised clinical trial: dried plums (prunes) vs. psyllium for constipation. *Aliment Pharmacol Ther.* 2011 Apr;33(7):822–8.

34. Enck P. Biofeedback training in disordered defecation: a critical review. *Dig Dis Sci.* 1993;38:1953–60.

Uncover secret problem foods

1. Simrén M, Månsson A, Langkilde AM, Svedlund J, Abrahamsson H,

Bengtsson U, Björnsson ES. Food-related gastrointestinal symptoms in the irritable bowel syndrome. *Digestion*. 2001;63(2):108–15.

2. Heizer WD, Southern S, McGovern S. The role of diet in symptoms of irritable bowel syndrome in adults: a narrative review. *J Am Diet Assoc*. 2009 Jul;109(7):1204–14.

3. Heizer WD, Southern S, McGovern S. The role of diet in symptoms of irritable bowel syndrome in adults: a narrative review. *J Am Diet Assoc*. 2009 Jul;109(7):1204–14.

4. Green PH, Cellier C. Celiac Disease. *N Engl J Med*. 2007;357:1731–43.

5. Presutti RJ, Cangemi JR, Cassidy HD, Hill DA. Celiac disease. *Am Fam Physician*. 2007 Dec 15;76(12):1795–802.

6. D'Amico MA, Holmes J, Stavropoulos SN, et al. Presentation of pediatric celiac disease in the United States: prominent effect of breastfeeding. *Clin Pediatr (Phila)*. 2005;44:249–58.

7. Presutti RJ, Cangemi JR, Cassidy HD, Hill DA. Celiac disease. *Am Fam Physician*. 2007 Dec 15;76(12):1795–802.

8. Niewinski MM. Advances in celiac disease and gluten-free diet. *J Am Diet Assoc*. 2008 Apr;108(4):661–72.

9. Green PH. The many faces of celiac disease: clinical presentation of celiac disease in the adult population. *Gastroenterology*. 2005 Apr;128(4 Suppl 1):S74–8.

10. Ford AC, Chey WD, Talley NJ, Malhotra A, Spiegel BM, Moayyedi P. Yield of diagnostic tests for celiac disease in individuals with symptoms suggestive of irritable bowel syndrome: systematic review and meta-analysis. *Arch Intern Med*. 2009 Apr 13;169(7):651–8.

11. American College of Gastroenterology Task Force on Irritable Bowel Syndrome, Brandt LJ, Chey WD, Foxx-Orenstein AE, Schiller LR, Schoenfeld PS, Spiegel BM, Talley NJ, Quigley EM. An evidence-based position statement on the management of irritable bowel syndrome. *Am J Gastroenterol*. 2009 Jan;104 Suppl 1:S1–35.

12. Niewinski MM. Advances in celiac disease and gluten-free diet. *J Am Diet Assoc*. 2008 Apr;108(4):661–72.

13. Biesiekierski JR, Newnham ED, Irving PM, Barrett JS, Haines M, Doecke JD, Shepherd SJ, Muir JG, Gibson PR. Gluten causes gastrointestinal symptoms in subjects without celiac disease:

a double-blind randomized placebo-controlled trial. *Am J Gastroenterol.* 2011 Mar;106(3):508–14.

14. Shahbazkhani B, Forootan M, Merat S, Akbari MR, Nasserimoghadam S, Vahedi H, Malekzadeh R. Coeliac disease presenting with symptoms of irritable bowel syndrome. *Aliment Pharmacol Ther.* 2003 Jul 15;18(2):231–5.

15. Usai P, Manca R, Cuomo R, Lai MA, Boi MF. Effect of gluten-free diet and co-morbidity of irritable bowel syndrome-type symptoms on health-related quality of life in adult coeliac patients. *Dig Liver Dis.* 2007 Sep;39(9):824–8.

16. Campbell AK, Matthews SB, Vassel N, Cox CD, Naseem R, Chaichi J, Holland IB, Green J, Wann KT. Bacterial metabolic 'toxins': a new mechanism for lactose and food intolerance, and irritable bowel syndrome. *Toxicology.* 2010 Dec 30;278(3):268–76.

17. Jellema P, Schellevis FG, van der Windt DA, Kneepkens CM, van der Horst HE. Lactose malabsorption and intolerance: a systematic review on the diagnostic value of gastrointestinal symptoms and self-reported milk intolerance. *QJM.* 2010 Aug;103(8):555–72.

18. Matthews SB, Waud JP, Roberts AG, Campbell AK. Systemic lactose intolerance: a new perspective on an old problem. *Postgrad Med J.* 2005 Mar;81(953):167–73.

19. Lomer MC, Parkes GC, Sanderson JD. Review article: lactose intolerance in clinical practice — myths and realities. *Aliment Pharmacol Ther.* 2008 Jan 15;27(2):93–103.

20. Rana SV, Mandal AK, Kochhar R, Katyal R, Singh K. Lactose intolerance in different types of irritable bowel syndrome in north Indians. *Trop Gastroenterol.* 2001 Oct–Dec;22(4):202–4.

21. Hertzler SR, Huynh BC, Savaiano DA. How much lactose is low lactose? *J Am Diet Assoc.* 1996 Mar;96(3):243–6.

22. Matthews SB, Waud JP, Roberts AG, Campbell AK. Systemic lactose intolerance: a new perspective on an old problem. *Postgrad Med J.* 2005 Mar;81(953):167–73.

23. Vernia P, Ricciardi MR, Frandina C, Bilotta T, Frieri G. Lactose malabsorption and irritable bowel syndrome. Effect of a long-term lactose-free diet. *Ital J Gastroenterol.* 1995 Apr;27(3):117–21.

24. Böhmer CJ, Tuynman HA. The effect of a lactose-restricted diet in patients with a positive lactose tolerance test, earlier diagnosed

as irritable bowel syndrome: a 5-year follow-up study. *Eur J Gastroenterol Hepatol.* 2001 Aug;13(8):941–4.

25. Crittenden RG, Bennett LE. Cow's milk allergy: a complex disorder. *J Am Coll Nutr.* 2005 Dec;24(6 Suppl):582S–91S.

26. Niec AM, Frankum B, Talley NJ. Are adverse food reactions linked to irritable bowel syndrome? *Am J Gastroenterol.* 1998 Nov;93(11):2184–90.

27. Atkinson W, Sheldon TA, Shaath N, Whorwell PJ. Food elimination based on IgG antibodies in irritable bowel syndrome: a randomised controlled trial. *Gut.* 2004 Oct;53(10):1459–64.

28. Zar S, Mincher L, Benson MJ, Kumar D. Food-specific IgG4 antibody-guided exclusion diet improves symptoms and rectal compliance in irritable bowel syndrome. *Scand J Gastroenterol.* 2005 Jul;40(7): 800–7.

29. Drisko J, Bischoff B, Hall M, McCallum R. Treating irritable bowel syndrome with a food elimination diet followed by food challenge and probiotics. *J Am Coll Nutr.* 2006 Dec;25(6):514–22.

30. Guo H, Jiang T, Wang J, Chang Y, Guo H, Zhang W. The value of eliminating foods according to food-specific immunoglobulin G antibodies in irritable bowel syndrome with diarrhoea. *J Int Med Res.* 2012;40(1):204–10.

31. Lerner A, Matthias T. Changes in intestinal tight junction permeability associated with industrial food additives explain the rising incidence of autoimmune disease. *Autoimmun Rev.* 2015 Jun;14(6):479–89.

32. Suez J, Korem T, Zeevi D, et al. Artificial sweeteners induce glucose intolerance by altering the gut microbiota. *Nature.* 2014 Oct 9;514(7521):181–6.

33. Abou-Donia MB, El-Masry EM, Abdel-Rahman AA, et al. Splenda alters gut microflora and increases intestinal p-glycoprotein and cytochrome p-450 in male rats. *J Toxicol Environ Health A.* 2008;71(21):1415–29.

34. Potera C. POPs and gut microbiota: dietary exposure alters ratio of bacterial species. *Environ Health Perspect.* 2015 Jul 1;123(7):A187.

35. Chassaing B, Koren O, Goodrich JK, et al. Dietary emulsifiers impact the mouse gut microbiota promoting colitis and metabolic syndrome. *Nature.* 2015 Mar 5;519(7541):92–6.

36. Nickerson KP, Chanin R, McDonald C. Deregulation of intestinal anti-microbial defense by the dietary additive, maltodextrin. *Gut Microbes.* 2015;6(1):78–83.

37. Holton KF, Taren DL, Thomson CA, Bennett RM, Jones KD. The effect of dietary glutamate on fibromyalgia and irritable bowel symptoms. *Clin Exp Rheumatol.* 2012 Nov-Dec;30(6 Suppl 74):10–7.

38. Maintz L, Novak N. Histamine and histamine intolerance. *Am J Clin Nutr.* 2007 May;85(5):1185–96.

39. Amon U, Bangha E, Küster T, Menne A, Vollrath IB, Gibbs BF. Enteral histaminosis: clinical implications. *Inflamm Res.* 1999 Jun;48(6): 291–5.

40. Maintz L, Novak N. Histamine and histamine intolerance. *Am J Clin Nutr.* 2007 May;85(5):1185–96.

41. Maintz L, et al. Histamine Intolerance, in *Clinical Practice.* Dtsch Arztebl 2006; 103(51–52): A 3477–83 [English translation].

42. Kohn JB. Is there a diet for histamine intolerance? *J Acad Nutr Diet.* 2014 Nov;114(11):1860.

43. Rosell-Camps A, Zibetti S, Pérez-Esteban G, et al. Histamine intolerance as a cause of chronic digestive complaints in pediatric patients. *Rev Esp Enferm Dig.* 2013 Apr;105(4):201–6.

44. Schwelberger HG. Histamine intolerance: a metabolic disease? *Inflamm Res.* 2010 Mar;59 Suppl 2:S219–21.

45. García-Martin E, Mendoza JL, Martínez C, et al. Severity of ulcerative colitis is associated with a polymorphism at diamine oxidase gene but not at histamine N-methyltransferase gene. *World J Gastroenterol.* 2006 Jan 28;12(4):615–20.

46. Szczepankiewicz A, Bręborowicz A, Sobkowiak P, Popiel A. Polymorphisms of two histamine-metabolizing enzymes genes and childhood allergic asthma: a case control study. *Clin Mol Allergy.* 2010 Nov 1;8:14.

47. García-Martín E, García-Menaya J, Sánchez B, Martínez C, Rosendo

R, Agúndez JA. Polymorphisms of histamine-metabolizing enzymes and clinical manifestations of asthma and allergic rhinitis. *Clin Exp Allergy.* 2007 Aug;37(8):1175–82.

48. García-Martín E, Martínez C, Serrador M, et al. Diamine oxidasers10156191 and rs2052129 variants are associated with the risk for migraine. *Headache.* 2015 Feb;55(2):276–86.

49. Spencer M, Chey WD, Eswaran S. Dietary renaissance in IBS: has food replaced medications as a primary treatment strategy? *Curr Treat Options Gastroenterol.* 2014 Dec;12(4):424–40.

50. Schwelberger HG. Histamine intolerance: overestimated or underestimated? *Inflamm Res.* 2009 Apr;58 suppl 1:51–2.

51. Wantke F, Götz M, Jarisch R. The histamine-free diet. *Hautarzt.* 1993 Aug;44(8):512–6.

52. Wantke F, Götz M, Jarisch R. Histamine-free diet: treatment of choice for histamine-induced food intolerance and supporting treatment for chronic headaches. *Clin Exp Allergy.* 1993 Dec;23(12):982–5.

53. Maintz L, Benfadal S, Allam JP, Hagemann T, Fimmers R, Novak N. Evidence for a reduced histamine degradation capacity in a subgroup of patients with atopic eczema. *J Allergy Clin Immunol.* 2006 May;117(5):1106–12.

54. Chung BY, Cho SI, Ahn IS, Lee HB, Kim HO, Park CW, Lee CH. Treatment of atopic dermatitis with a low-histamine diet. *Ann Dermatol.* 2011 Sep;23 suppl 1:S91-5. doi: 10.5021/ad.2011.23.S1.S91.

55. Hoffmann KM, Gruber E, Deutschmann A, Jahnel J, Hauer AC. Histamine intolerance in children with chronic abdominal pain. *Arch Dis Child.* 2013 Oct;98(10):832–3.

56. Rosell-Camps A, Zibetti S, Pérez-Esteban G, et al. Histamine intolerance as a cause of chronic digestive complaints in pediatric patients. *Rev Esp Enferm Dig.* 2013 Apr;105(4):201–6.

57. Wouters MM, Balemans D, Van Wanrooy S, et al. Histamine receptor H1-mediated sensitization of TRPV1 mediates visceral hypersensitivity and symptoms in patients with irritable bowel syndrome. *Gastroenterology.* 2016 Apr;150(4):875–87.e9.

58. Fasano A, Catassi C. Clinical practice. Celiac disease. *N Engl J Med.* 2012 Dec 20;367(25):2419–26.

59. Johnston CS, Martin LJ, Cai X. Antihistamine effect of supplemental ascorbic acid and neutrophil chemotaxis. *J Am Coll Nutr.* 1992 Apr;11(2):172–6.

60. Martner-Hewes PM, Hunt IF, Murphy NJ, Swendseid ME, Settlage RH. Vitamin B-6 nutriture and plasma diamine oxidase activity in pregnant Hispanic teenagers. *Am J Clin Nutr.* 1986 Dec;44(6): 907–13.

61. Oksaharju A, Kankainen M, Kekkonen RA, et al. Probiotic Lactobacillus rhamnosus downregulates FCER1 and HRH4 expression in human mast cells. *World J Gastroenterol.* 2011 Feb 14;17(6):750–9.

Put your bacteria on a low-carbohydrate diet

1. Beyer PL, Caviar EM, McCallum RW. Fructose intake at current levels in the United States may cause gastrointestinal distress in normal adults. *J Am Diet Assoc.* 2005;105: 1559–66.

2. Hurst A, Knott F. Intestinal carbohydrate dyspepsia. *QJM.* Jan 1931; 94:171–9.

3. Kneepkens CM, Vonk RJ, Fernandes J. Incomplete intestinal absorption of fructose. *Arch Dis Child.* 1984 Aug;59(8):735–8.

4. Andersson DE, Nygren A. Four cases of longstanding diarrhoea and colic pains cured by fructose-free diet — a pathogenetic discussion. *Acta Med Scand.* 1978;203:87–92.

5. Ledochowski M, Widner B, Bair H, et al. Fructose- and sorbitol-reduced diet improves mood and gastrointestinal disturbances in fructose malabsorbers. *Scand J Gastroenterol.* 2000;35:1048–52.

6. Bray GA. Fructose: pure, white, and deadly? Fructose, by any other name, is a health hazard. *J Diabetes Sci Technol.* 2010 Jul 1;4(4):1003–7.

7. Marriott BP, Cole N, Lee E. National estimates of dietary fructose intake increased from 1977 to 2004 in the United States. *J Nutr.* 2009 Jun;139(6):1228S–1235S.

8. Park YK, Yetley EA. Intakes and food sources of fructose in the United States. *Am J Clin Nutr.* 1993 Nov;58(5 Suppl):737S–747S.

9. Beyer PL, Caviar EM, McCallum RW. Fructose intake at current levels in the United States may cause gastrointestinal distress in normal adults. *J Am Diet Assoc.* 2005 Oct; 105(10):1559–66.

10. Gibson PR, Newnham E, Barrett JS, Shepherd SJ, Muir JG. Review article: fructose malabsorption and the bigger picture. *Aliment Pharmacol Ther*. 2007 Feb 15;25(4):349–63.

11. Latulippe ME, Skoog SM. Fructose malabsorption and intolerance: effects of fructose with and without simultaneous glucose ingestion. *Crit Rev Food Sci Nutr*. 2011 Aug;51(7):583–92.

12. Rumessen JJ, Gudmand-Høyer E. Malabsorption of fructose-sorbitol mixtures. Interactions causing abdominal distress. *Scand J Gastroenterol*. 1987;22:431–6.

13. Walker ARP, Segal I. Epidemiology of noninfective intestinal diseases in various ethnic groups in Southern Africa. Israel J Med Sci 1979;15: 309–13.

14. Bijkerk CJ, Muris JW, Knottnerus JA, Hoes AW, de Wit NJ. Systematic review: the role of different types of fibre in the treatment of irritable bowel syndrome. *Aliment Pharmacol Ther*. 2004 Feb 1;19(3):245–51.

15. Nanda R, James R, Smith H, Dudley CR, Jewell DP. Food intolerance and the irritable bowel syndrome. *Gut*. 1989;30:1099–104.

16. Dear KLE, Elia M, Hunter JO. Do interventions which reduce colonic bacterial fermentation improve symptoms of irritable bowel syndrome? *Dig Dis Sci*. 2005;50:758–66.

17. King TS, Elia M, Hunter JO. Abnormal colonic fermentation in irritable bowel syndrome. *Lancet*. 1998;352:1187–9.

18. Goldstein R, Braverman D, Stankiewicz H. Carbohydrate malabsorption and the effect of dietary restriction on symptoms of irritable bowel syndrome and functional bowel complaints. *Isr Med Assoc J*. 2000;2:583–7.

19. Austin GL, Dalton CB, Hu Y, Morris CB, Hankins J, Weinland SR, Westman EC, Yancy WS Jr, Drossman DA. A very low-carbohydrate diet improves symptoms and quality of life in diarrhoea-predominant irritable bowel syndrome. *Clin Gastroenterol Hepatol*. 2009 Jun;7(6):706–708.e1.

20. Bijkerk CJ, Muris JW, Knottnerus JA, Hoes AW, de Wit NJ. Systematic review: the role of different types of fibre in the treatment of irritable bowel syndrome. *Aliment Pharmacol Ther*. 2004 Feb 1;19(3):245–51.

21. Staudacher HM, Whelan K, Irving PM, Lomer MC. Comparison of symptom response following advice for a diet low in fermentable carbohydrates (FODMAPs) versus standard dietary advice in patients with irritable bowel syndrome. *J Hum Nutr Diet*. 2011 Oct;24(5):487–95.

22. Barrett JS, Gearry RB, Muir JG, Irving PM, Rose R, Rosella O, Haines ML, Shepherd SJ, Gibson PR. Dietary poorly absorbed, short-chain carbohydrates increase delivery of water and fermentable substrates to the proximal colon. *Aliment Pharmacol Ther*. 2010 Apr;31(8):874–82.

23. Gibson PR, Shepherd SJ. Personal view: food for thought — western lifestyle and susceptibility to Crohn's disease. The FODMAP hypothesis. *Aliment Pharmacol Ther*. 2005 Jun 15;21(12):1399–409.

24. Barrett JS, Irving PM, Shepherd SJ, Muir JG, Gibson PR. Comparison of the prevalence of fructose and lactose malabsorption across chronic intestinal disorders. *Aliment Pharmacol Ther*. 2009 Jul 1;30(2): 165–74.

25. Ierardi E, Losurdo G, Sorrentino C, et al. Macronutrient intakes in obese subjects with or without small intestinal bacterial overgrowth: an alimentary survey. *Scand J Gastroenterol*. 2016 Mar;51(3):277–80.

26. Nucera G, Gabrielli M, Lupascu A, Lauritano EC, Santoliquido A, Cremonini F, Cammarota G, Tondi P, Pola P, Gasbarrini G, Gasbarrini A. Abnormal breath tests to lactose, fructose and sorbitol in irritable bowel syndrome may be explained by small intestinal bacterial overgrowth. *Aliment Pharmacol Ther*. 2005 Jun 1;21(11):1391–5.

27. Böhn L, et al. Diet low in FODMAPs reduces symptoms of irritable bowel syndrome as well as traditional dietary advice: a randomized controlled trial. *Gastroenterology*. 2015 Aug 5. pii: S0016-5085(15)01086-0.

28. Haas SV, Haas MP. The treatment of celiac disease with the Specific Carbohydrate Diet; report on 191 additional cases. *Am J Gastroenterol*. 1955 Apr;23(4):344–60.

29. Gottschall E. *Breaking the Vicious Cycle: Intestinal health through diet*. Baltimore, Canada: Kirkton Press; 1987.

30. Walters SSQA, Rolston M. Analysis of gut microbiome and diet modification in patients with Crohn's disease. *SOJ Microbiol Infect Dis*. 2014;2:1–13.

31. Kakodkar S, Farooqui AJ, Mikolaitis SL, Mutlu EA. The Specific Carbohydrate Diet for Inflammatory Bowel Disease: a case series. *J Acad Nutr Diet.* 2015 Aug;115(8):1226–32.

32. Obih C, Wahbeh G, Lee D, Braly K, Giefer M, Shaffer ML, Nielson H, Suskind DL. Specific Carbohydrate Diet for pediatric Inflammatory Bowel Disease in clinical practice within an academic IBD center. *Nutrition.* 2015 Nov 30. pii: S0899-9007(15)00389–5.

33. Suskind DL, Wahbeh G, Gregory N, Vendettuoli H, Christie D. Nutritional therapy in pediatric Crohn disease: the Specific Carbohydrate Diet. *J Pediatr Gastroenterol Nutr.* 2014 Jan;58(1): 87–91.

34. Khandalavala BN, Nirmalraj MC. Resolution of severe ulcerative colitis with the Specific Carbohydrate Diet. *Case Rep Gastroenterol.* 2015 Aug 7;9(2):291–5.

35. Cohen SA, Gold BD, Oliva S, Lewis J, Stallworth A, Koch B, Eshee L, Mason D. Clinical and mucosal improvement with Specific Carbohydrate Diet in pediatric Crohn disease. J Pediatr Gastroenterol Nutr. 2014 Oct;59(4):516–21.

36. O'Dwyer DD, Darville RL. Specific Carbohydrate Diet: irritable bowel syndrome patient case study. *Nutrition & Food Science.* 2015 vol. 45 Iss: 6, pp.859–72.

Rewire the nerves of your gut–brain axis

1. Spiller R, Aziz Q, Creed F, Emmanuel A, Houghton L, Hungin P, Jones R, Kumar D, Rubin G, Trudgill N, Whorwell P; Clinical Services Committee of The British Society of Gastroenterology. Guidelines on the irritable bowel syndrome: mechanisms and practical management. *Gut.* 2007 Dec;56(12):1770–98.

2. Chitkara DK, van Tilburg MA, Blois-Martin N, Whitehead WE. Early life risk factors that contribute to irritable bowel syndrome in adults: a systematic review. *Am J Gastroenterol.* 2008 Mar;103(3):765–74.

3. Koloski NA, Jones M, Kalantar J, Weltman M, Zaguirre J, Talley NJ. The brain–gut pathway in functional gastrointestinal disorders is bidirectional: a 12-year prospective population-based study. *Gut.* 2012 Jan 10. [Epub ahead of print]

4. Ford MJ, Miller PM, Eastwood J, Eastwood MA. Life events, psychiatric illness and the irritable bowel syndrome. *Gut.* 1987 Feb;28(2):160–5.

5. Bennett EJ, Tennant CC, Piesse C, Badcock CA, Kellow JE. Level of chronic life stress predicts clinical outcome in irritable bowel syndrome. *Gut*. 1998 Aug;43(2):256–61.

6. McEwen BS. Protective and damaging effects of stress mediators. *N Engl J Med*. 1998 Jan 15;338(3):171–9.

7. Tsigos C, Chrousos GP. Hypothalamic-pituitary-adrenal axis, neuroendocrine factors and stress. *J Psychosom Res*. 2002 Oct;53(4):865–71.

8. Kudielka BM, Hellhammer DH, Wüst S. Why do we respond so differently? Reviewing determinants of human salivary cortisol responses to challenge. *Psychoneuroendocrinology*. 2009 Jan;34(1):2–18.

9. Tsigos C, Chrousos GP. Hypothalamic-pituitary-adrenal axis, neuroendocrine factors and stress. *J Psychosom Res*. 2002 Oct;53(4):865–71.

10. Chang L, Sundaresh S, Elliott J, Anton PA, Baldi P, Licudine A, Mayer M, Vuong T, Hirano M, Naliboff BD, Ameen VZ, Mayer EA. Dysregulation of the hypothalamic-pituitary-adrenal (HPA) axis in irritable bowel syndrome. *Neurogastroenterol Motil*. 2009 Feb;21(2):149–59.

11. Dinan TG, Quigley EM, Ahmed SM, Scully P, O'Brien S, O'Mahony L, O'Mahony S, Shanahan F, Keeling PW. Hypothalamic-pituitary-gut axis dysregulation in irritable bowel syndrome: plasma cytokines as a potential biomarker? *Gastroenterology*. 2006 Feb;130(2):304–11.

12. Heitkemper MM, Cain KC, Deechakawan W, Poppe A, Jun SE, Burr RL, Jarrett ME. Anticipation of public speaking and sleep and the hypothalamic-pituitary-adrenal axis in women with irritable bowel syndrome. *Neurogastroenterol Motil*. 2012 Jul;24(7):626-e271.

13. Murray CD, Flynn J, Ratcliffe L, Jacyna MR, Kamm MA, Emmanuel AV. Effect of acute physical and psychological stress on gut autonomic innervation in irritable bowel syndrome. *Gastroenterology*. 2004 Dec;127(6):1695–703.

14. Mayer EA, Tillisch K. The brain–gut axis in abdominal pain syndromes. *Annu Rev Med*. 2011;62:381–96.

15. Tillisch K, Mayer EA, Labus JS. Quantitative meta-analysis identifies brain regions activated during rectal distention in irritable bowel syndrome. *Gastroenterology.* 2011 Jan;140(1):91–100.

16. Lyte M, Varcoe JJ, Bailey MT. Anxiogenic effect of subclinical bacterial infection in mice in the absence of overt immune activation. *Physiol Behav.* 1998 Aug;65(1):63–8.

17. Bercik P, Park AJ, Sinclair D, Khoshdel A, Lu J, Huang X, Deng Y, Blennerhassett PA, Fahnestock M, Moine D, Berger B, Huizinga JD, Kunze W, McLean PG, Bergonzelli GE, Collins SM, Verdu EF. The anxiolytic effect of Bifidobacterium longum NCC3001 involves vagal pathways for gut-brain communication. *Neurogastroenterol Motil.* 2011 Dec;23(12):1132–9.

18. Messaoudi M, Lalonde R, Violle N, Javelot H, Desor D, Nejdi A, Bisson JF, Rougeot C, Pichelin M, Cazaubiel M, Cazaubiel JM. Assessment of psychotropic-like properties of a probiotic formulation (Lactobacillus helveticus R0052 and Bifidobacterium longum R0175) in rats and human subjects. *Br J Nutr.* 2011 Mar;105(5):755–64.

19. Lackner JM, Jaccard J, Krasner SS, Katz LA, Gudleski GD, Blanchard EB. How does cognitive behavior therapy for irritable bowel syndrome work? A mediational analysis of a randomized clinical trial. *Gastroenterology.* 2007 Aug; 133(2):433–44.

20. Lackner JM, Lou Coad M, Mertz HR, Wack DS, Katz LA, Krasner SS, Firth R, Mahl TC, Lockwood AH. Cognitive therapy for irritable bowel syndrome is associated with reduced limbic activity, GI symptoms, and anxiety. *Behav Res Ther.* 2006 May;44(5):621–38.

21. Lackner JM, Jaccard J, Krasner SS, Katz LA, Gudleski GD, Holroyd K. Self-administered cognitive behavior therapy for moderate to severe irritable bowel syndrome: clinical efficacy, tolerability, feasibility. *Clin Gastroenterol Hepatol.* 2008 Aug;6(8):899–906.

22. Whitehead WE. Hypnosis for irritable bowel syndrome: the empirical evidence of therapeutic effects. *Int J Clin Exp Hypn.* 2006 Jan;54(1):7–20.

Reset your digestive clock

1. Luscombe FA. Health-related quality of life and associated psychosocial factors in irritable bowel syndrome: a review. *Qual Life Res.* 2000;9:161–76.

2. Elsenbruch S, Thompson JJ, Hamish MJ, et al. Behavioral and physiological sleep characteristics in women with irritable bowel syndrome. *Am J Gastroenterol* 2002;97:2306–14.

3. Goldsmith G, Levin JS. Effect of sleep quality on symptoms of irritable bowel syndrome. *Dig Dis Sci.* 1993 Oct;38(10):1809–14.

4. Cremonini F, Camilleri M, Zinsmeister AR, Herrick LM, Beebe T, Talley NJ. Sleep disturbances are linked to both upper and lower gastrointestinal symptoms in the general population. *Neurogastroenterol Motil.* 2009 Feb;21(2):128–35.

5. Nojkov B, Rubenstein JH, Chey WD, Hoogerwerf WA. The impact of rotating shift work on the prevalence of irritable bowel syndrome in nurses. *Am J Gastroenterol.* 2010 Apr;105(4):842–7.

6. Onen SH, Alloui A, Gross A, Eschallier A, Dubray C. The effects of total sleep deprivation, selective sleep interruption and sleep recovery on pain tolerance thresholds in healthy subjects. *J Sleep Res.* 2001 Mar;10(1):35–42.

7. Roehrs T, Hyde M, Blaisdell B, Greenwald M, Roth T. Sleep loss and REM sleep loss are hyperalgesic. *Sleep.* 2006 Feb;29(2):145–51.

8. van Geijlswijk IM, Korzilius HP, Smits MG. The use of exogenous melatonin in delayed sleep phase disorder: a meta-analysis. *Sleep.* 2010 Dec;33(12):1605–14.

9. Chen CQ, Fichna J, Bashashati M, Li YY, Storr M. Distribution, function and physiological role of melatonin in the lower gut. *World J Gastroenterol.* 2011 Sep 14;17(34):3888–98.

10. Roberts-Thomson IC, Knight RE, Kennaway DJ, et al. Circadian rhythms in patients with abdominal pain syndromes. *Aust NZ J Med*, 1988;18:569–74.

11. 11. Song GH, Leng PH, Gwee KA, et al. Melatonin improves abdominal pain in irritable bowel syndrome patients who have sleep disturbances: a randomised, double blind, placebo controlled study. *Gut*. 2005;54:1402–7.

12. Lu WZ, Gwee KA, Moochhalla S, Ho KY. Melatonin improves bowel symptoms in female patients with irritable bowel syndrome: a double-blind placebo-controlled study. *Aliment Pharmacol Ther*. 2005 Nov 15;22(10):927–34.

13. Saha L, Malhotra S, Rana S, Bhasin D, Pandhi P. A preliminary study of melatonin in irritable bowel syndrome. *J Clin Gastroenterol*. 2007 Jan;41(1):29–32.

14. Mirick DK, Davis S. Melatonin as a biomarker of circadian dyoregulation. *Cancer Epidemiol Biomarkers Prev*. 2008 Dec, 17(12):3306–13.

15. Lewy AJ, Wehr TA, Goodwin FK, Newsome DA, Markey SP. Light suppresses melatonin secretion in humans. *Science*. 1980;210:1267–69.

16. Zeitzer JM, Dijk DJ, Kronauer R, et al. Sensitivity of the human circadian pacemaker to nocturnal light: melatonin phase resetting and suppression. *J Physiol*. 2000;526 Pt 3:695–702.

17. Buckley TM, Schatzberg AF. On the interactions of the hypothalamic-pituitary-adrenal (HPA) axis and sleep: normal HPA axis activity and circadian rhythm, exemplary sleep disorders. *J Clin Endocrinol Metab*. 2005 May;90(5):3106–14.

18. Kumar D, Thompson PD, Wingate DL, Vesselinova-Jenkins CK, Libby G. Abnormal REM sleep in the irritable bowel syndrome. *Gastroenterology*. 1992 Jul;103(1):12–7.

19. Malhotra S, Sawhney G, Pandhi P. The therapeutic potential of melatonin: a review of the science. *MedGenMed*. 2004 Apr 13;6(2):46.

Get on a digestive fitness program

1. Booth FW, Laye MJ, Lees SJ, Rector RS, Thyfault JP. Reduced physical activity and risk of chronic disease: the biology behind the consequences. *Eur J Appl Physiol.* 2008 Mar;102(4):381-90.

2. Martin D. Physical activity benefits and risks on the gastrointestinal system. *South Med J.* 2011 Dec;104(12):831-7.

3. O'Keefe JH, Vogel R, Lavie CJ, Cordain L. Achieving hunter-gatherer fitness in the 21(st) century: back to the future. *Am J Med.* 2010 Dec;123(12):1082-6.

4. Booth FW, Lees SJ. Fundamental questions about genes, inactivity, and chronic diseases. *Physiol Genomics.* 2007 Jan 17;28(2):146-57.

5. Colwell LJ, Prather CM, Phillips SF, Zinsmeister AR. Effects of an irritable bowel syndrome educational class on health-promoting behaviors and symptoms. *Am J Gastroenterol.* 1998 Jun;93(6):901-5.

6. Lustyk MK, Jarrett ME, Bennett JC, Heitkemper MM. Does a physically active lifestyle improve symptoms in women with irritable bowel syndrome? *Gastroenterol Nurs.* 2001 May-Jun;24(3):129-37. PubMed PMID: 11847862.

7. Daley AJ, Grimmett C, Roberts L, Wilson S, Fatek M, Roalfe A, Singh S. The effects of exercise upon symptoms and quality of life in patients diagnosed with irritable bowel syndrome: a randomised controlled trial. *Int J Sports Med.* 2008 Sep;29(9):778-82.

8. Johannesson E, Simrén M, Strid H, Bajor A, Sadik R. Physical activity improves symptoms in irritable bowel syndrome: a randomized controlled trial. *Am J Gastroenterol.* 2011 May;106(5):915-22.

9. Villoria A, Serra J, Azpiroz F, Malagelada JR. Physical activity and intestinal gas clearance in patients with bloating. *Am J Gastroenterol.* 2006 Nov;101(11):2552-7.

10. De Schryver AM, Keulemans YC, Peters HP, Akkermans LM, Smout AJ, De Vries WR, van Berge-Henegouwen GP. Effects of regular physical activity on defecation pattern in middle-aged patients complaining of chronic constipation. *Scand J Gastroenterol.* 2005 Apr;40(4):422-9.

11. Brands MM, Purperhart H, Deckers-Kocken JM. A pilot study of yoga treatment in children with functional abdominal pain and irritable bowel syndrome. *Complement Ther Med.* 2011 Jun;19(3):109–14.

12. Kuttner L, Chambers CT, Hardial J, Israel DM, Jacobson K, Evans K. A randomized trial of yoga for adolescents with irritable bowel syndrome. *Pain Res Manag.* 2006 Winter;11(4):217–23.

The five-step plan for digestive health

1. Grigoleit HG, Grigoleit P. Pharmacology and preclinical pharmacokinetics of peppermint oil. *Phytomedicine.* 2005 Aug;12(8):612–6.

2. Kingham JG. Peppermint oil and colon spasm. *Lancet* 346.8981 (1995): 986.

3. Grigoleit HG, Grigoleit P. Gastrointestinal clinical pharmacology of peppermint oil. *Phytomedicine.* 2005 Aug;12(8):607–11.

4. Braun L, Cohen M. *Herbs and Natural Supplements: An Evidence-Based Guide* 3rd edn. Churchill Livingstone, 2010.

5. Merat S, Khalili S, Mostajabi P, Ghorbani A, Ansari R, Malekzadeh R. The effect of enteric-coated, delayed-release peppermint oil on irritable bowel syndrome. *Dig Dis Sci.* 2010 May;55(5):1385–90.

6. Kligler B, Chaudhary S. Peppermint oil. *Am Fam Physician.* 2007 Apr 1;75(7):1027–30.

7. Suarez F, Levitt MD, Adshead J, Barkin JS. Pancreatic supplements reduce symptomatic response of healthy subjects to a high fat meal. *Dig Dis Sci.* 1999 Jul;44(7):1317–21.

8. Fieker A, Philpott J, Armand M. Enzyme replacement therapy for pancreatic insufficiency: present and future. *Clin Exp Gastroenterol.* 2011;4:55–73.

9. Emendörfer F, Emendörfer F, Bellato F, Noldin VF, Cechinel-Filho V, Yunes RA, Delle Monache F, Cardozo AM. Antispasmodic activity of fractions and cynaropicrin from Cynara scolymus on guinea-pig ileum. *Biol Pharm Bull.* 2005 May;28(5):902–4. PubMed PMID: 15863902.

10. Kirchhoff R, et al. Increase in cholesteresis by means of artichoke extract. *Phytomedicine.* 1994;1:107–15.

11. Walker AF, Middleton RW, Petrowicz O. Artichoke leaf extract reduces symptoms of irritable bowel syndrome in a post-marketing surveillance study. *Phytother Res.* 2001 Feb;15(1):58–61.

12. Bundy R, Walker AF, Middleton RW, Marakis G, Booth JC. Artichoke leaf extract reduces symptoms of irritable bowel syndrome and improves quality of life in otherwise healthy volunteers suffering from concomitant dyspepsia: a subset analysis. *J Altern Complement Med.* 2004 Aug;10(4):667–9.

13. Fintelmann V. Antidyspeptic and lipid-lowering effects of artichoke leaf extract: results of clinical studies into the efficacy and tolerance of Hepar-SL® forte involving 553 patients. *J Gen Med.* 1996;2:3–19.

14. Benzie IFF, Wachtel-Galor S, editors. *Herbal Medicine: Biomolecular and Clinical Aspects* 2nd edn. Boca Raton (FL): CRC Press, 2011.

15. Ottillinger B, Storr M, Malfertheiner P, Allescher HD. STW 5 (Iberogast®) — a safe and effective standard in the treatment of functional gastrointestinal disorders. *Wien Med Wochenschr.* 2013 Feb;163(3–4):65–72.

16. Oka T, Okumi H, Nishida S, Ito T, Morikiyo S, Kimura Y, Murakami M. Effects of Kampo on functional gastrointestinal disorders. *Biopsychosoc Med.* 2014 Jan 21;8(1):5.

17. 17. Bensoussan A, Talley NJ, Hing M, Menzies R, Guo A, Ngu M. Treatment of irritable bowel syndrome with Chinese herbal medicine: a randomized controlled trial. *JAMA.* 1998 Nov 11;280(18):1585–9.

18. 18. Bian Z, Wu T, Liu L, Miao J, Wong H, Song L, Sung JJ. Effectiveness of the Chinese herbal formula TongXieYaoFang for irritable bowel syndrome: a systematic review. *J Altern Complement Med.* 2006 May;12(4):401–7.

19. Sahib AS. Treatment of irritable bowel syndrome using a selected herbal combination of Iraqi folk medicines. *J Ethnopharmacol.* 2013 Jul 30;148(3):1008–12.

20. Wegener T, Wagner H. The active components and the pharmacological multi-target principle of STW 5 (Iberogast). *Phytomedicine.* 2006;13 Suppl 5:20–35.

21. Madisch A, Holtmann G, Plein K, Hotz J. Treatment of irritable bowel syndrome with herbal preparations: results of a double-blind, randomized, placebo-controlled, multi-centre trial. *Aliment Pharmacol Ther*. 2004 Feb 1;19(3): 271-9.

22. Mizuno S, Nagata K, Yoshida K, Sasaki H, Kojo H, Miura K, Tamura N, Hirayama S, Nakagawa T, Inoue M, Ogawa N: *Kabinsei Cho Shoukougun ni taisuru keishikashakuyakuto ekisu no chiryo kouka — mepenzolate bromide tono hikaku shiken* (Japanese). *Shindan to Chiryo*. 1985;73:1143-1152.

23. Ottillinger B, Storr M, Malfertheiner P, Allescher HD. STW 5 (Iberogast®) — a safe and effective standard in the treatment of functional gastrointestinal disorders. *Wien Med Wochenschr*. 2012 Dec 20. [Epub ahead of print]

24. Langmead L, Feakins RM, Goldthorpe S, Holt H, Tsironi E, De Silva A, Jewell DP, Rampton DS. Randomized, double-blind, placebo-controlled trial of oral aloe vera gel for active ulcerative colitis. *Aliment Pharmacol Ther*. 2004 Apr 1;19(7):739-47.

25. Bland J. Aloe vera juice: an important role in gastrointestinal disorders? *Altern Med 1*. 1986:280.

26. Davis K, Philpott S, Kumar D, Mendall M. Randomised double-blind placebo-controlled trial of aloe vera for irritable bowel syndrome. *Int J Clin Pract*. 2006 Sep;60(9):1080-6.

27. Khedmat H, Karbasi A, Amini M, et al. Aloe vera in treatment of refractory irritable bowel syndrome: trial on Iranian patients. *J Res Med Sci*. 2013 Aug;18(8):732.

28. DuPont AW, DuPont HL. The intestinal microbiota and chronic disorders of the gut. *Nat Rev Gastroenterol Hepatol*. 2011 Aug 16;8(9):523-31.

29. Almansa C, Agrawal A, Houghton LA. Intestinal microbiota, pathophysiology and translation to probiotic use in patients with irritable bowel syndrome. *Expert Rev Gastroenterol Hepatol*. 2012 Jun;6(3):383-98.

30. Clarke G, Cryan JF, Dinan TG, Quigley EM. Review article: probiotics for the treatment of irritable bowel syndrome — focus on lactic acid bacteria. *Aliment Pharmacol Ther*. 2012 Feb;35(4):403-13.

31. McKenzie YA, Alder A, Anderson W, Wills A, Goddard L, Gulia P, Jankovich E, Mutch P, Reeves LB, Singer A, Lomer MC; Gastroenterology Specialist Group of the British Dietetic Association. British Dietetic Association evidence-based guidelines for the dietary management of irritable bowel syndrome in adults. *J Hum Nutr Diet.* 2012 Jun;25(3):260–74.

32. Ducrotté P, et al. Clinical trial: *Lactobacillus plantarum* 299v (DSM 9843) improves symptoms of irritable bowel syndrome. *World J Gastroenterol.* 2012 Aug 14;18(30):4012–8.

33. Sen S, et al. Effect of *Lactobacillus plantarum* 299v on colonic fermentation and symptoms of irritable bowel syndrome. Dig Dis Sci. 2002 Nov;47(11):2615–20.

34. Niedzielin K, et al. A controlled, double-blind, randomized study on the efficacy of *Lactobacillus plantarum* 299V in patients with irritable bowel syndrome. *Eur J Gastroenterol Hepatol.* 2001 Oct;13(10):1143–7.

35. Whorwell PJ, et al. Efficacy of an encapsulated probiotic *Bifidobacterium infantis* 35624 in women with irritable bowel syndrome. *Am J Gastroenterol.* 2006 Jul;101(7):1581–90.

36. O'Mahony L, et al. *Lactobacillus* and *bifidobacterium* in irritable bowel syndrome: symptom responses and relationship to cytokine profiles. *Gastroenterology.* 2005 Mar;128(3):541–51.

37. Williams EA, et al. Clinical trial: a multi-strain probiotic preparation significantly reduces symptoms of irritable bowel syndrome in a double-blind placebo-controlled study. *Aliment Pharmacol Ther.* 2009 Jan;29(1):97–103.

38. Enck P, et al Randomized controlled treatment trial of irritable bowel syndrome with a probiotic *E.-coli* preparation (DSM17252) compared to placebo. *Z Gastroenterol.* 2009 Feb;47(2):209–14.

39. Enck P, et al. A mixture of *Escherichia coli* (DSM 17252) and *Enterococcus faecalis* (DSM 16440) for treatment of the irritable bowel syndrome — a randomized controlled trial with primary care physicians. *Neurogastroenterol Motil.* 2008 Oct;20(10):1103–9.

40. Martens U, et al. Probiotic treatment of irritable bowel syndrome in children. *Ger Med Sci.* 2010 Mar 2;8:Doc07.

41. Guandalini S, et al. VSL#3 improves symptoms in children with irritable bowel syndrome: a multicenter, randomized, placebo-controlled, double-blind, crossover study. *J Pediatr Gastroenterol Nutr.* 2010 Jul;51(1):24–30.

42. Kim HJ, et al. A randomized controlled trial of a probiotic combination VSL# 3 and placebo in irritable bowel syndrome with bloating. *Neurogastroenterol Motil.* 2005 Oct;17(5):687–96.

43. Kim HJ, et al. A randomized controlled trial of a probiotic, VSL#3, on gut transit and symptoms in diarrhoea-predominant irritable bowel syndrome. *Aliment Pharmacol Ther.* 2003 Apr 1;17(7):895–904.

44. Abbas Z, et al. Cytokine and clinical response to *Saccharomyces boulardii* therapy in diarrhea-dominant irritable bowel syndrome: a randomized trial. *Eur J Gastroenterol Hepatol.* 2014 Jun,26(6). 630–9.

45. Choi CH, et al. A randomized, double-blind, placebo-controlled multicenter trial of *Saccharomyces boulardii* in irritable bowel syndrome: effect on quality of life. *J Clin Gastroenterol.* 2011; 45: 679–83.

46. Maupas, J, et al. Treatment of irritable bowel syndrome with *Saccharomyces boulardii*: a double-blind, placebo-controlled-study. *Med Chir Dig.* 1983;12, 77–9.

47. Kabir MA, et al. Role of *Saccharomyces boulardii* in diarrhea predominant irritable bowel syndrome. *Mymensingh Med J.* 2011; 20: 97–401.

48. Pineton de Chambrun G, Neut C, Chau A, et al. A randomized clinical trial of *Saccharomyces cerevisiae* versus placebo in the irritable bowel syndrome. *Dig Liver Dis.* 2015 Feb;47(2):119–24.

49. Dolin BJ. Effects of a proprietary *Bacillus coagulans* preparation on symptoms of diarrhea-predominant irritable bowel syndrome. *Methods Find Exp Clin Pharmacol.* 2009 Dec;31(10):655–9.

50. Hun L. Bacillus coagulans significantly improved abdominal pain and bloating in patients with IBS. *Postgrad Med.* 2009 Mar;121(2):119–24.

51. Zhang Y, Li L, Guo C, et al. Effects of probiotic type, dose and treatment duration on irritable bowel syndrome diagnosed by Rome III criteria: a meta-analysis. *BMC Gastroenterol.* 2016 Jun 13;16(1):62.

52. Shah, NP, et al., 1995. Survival of Lactobacillus acidophilus and Bifidobacterium bifidum in commercial yoghurt during refrigerated storage. *International Dairy Journal*. 5, 515–21.

53. del Campo R, et al. Scarce evidence of yogurt lactic acid bacteria in human feces after daily yogurt consumption by healthy volunteers. *Appl Environ Microbiol*. 2005;71:547–9.

54. McKenzie YA, Alder A, Anderson W, et al; Gastroenterology Specialist Group of the British Dietetic Association. British Dietetic Association evidence-based guidelines for the dietary management of irritable bowel syndrome in adults. *J Hum Nutr Diet*. 2012 Jun;25(3):260–74.

55. Yazawa K, Imai K & Tamura Z. Oligosaccharides and polysaccharides specifically utilizable by bifidobacteria. *Chem Pharm Bull* 1978;26:3306–11.

56. Silk DB, Davis A, Vulevic J, Tzortzis G, Gibson GR. Clinical trial: the effects of a trans-galactooligosaccharide prebiotic on faecal microbiota and symptoms in irritable bowel syndrome. *Aliment Pharmacol Ther*. 2009 Mar 1;29(5):508–18.

57. Paineau D, Payen F, Panserieu S, et al. The effects of regular consumption of short-chain fructo-oligosaccharides on digestive comfort of subjects with minor functional bowel disorders. *Br J Nutr*. 2008;99:311–318.

58. Roberfroid M, Gibson GR, Hoyles L et al. Prebiotic effects: metabolic and health benefits. *Br J Nutr*. 2010 Aug;104 Suppl 2:S1–63.

59. Brown K, DeCoffe D, Molcan E, Gibson DL. Diet-induced dysbiosis of the intestinal microbiota and the effects on immunity and disease. *Nutrients*. 2012 Aug;4(8):1095–119.

60. Shinohara K, Ohashi Y, Kawasumi K, Terada A, Fujisawa T. Effect of apple intake on fecal microbiota and metabolites in humans. *Anaerobe*. 2010 Oct;16(5):510–5.

61. Mitsou EK, Kougia E, Nomikos T, Yannakoulia M, Mountzouris KC, Kyriacou A. Effect of banana consumption on faecal microbiota: a randomised, controlled trial. *Anaerobe*. 2011 Dec;17(6):384–7.

62. Vendrame S, Guglielmetti S, Riso P, Arioli S, Klimis-Zacas D, Porrini M. Six-week consumption of a wild blueberry powder drink increases bifidobacteria in the human gut. *J Agric Food Chem*. 2011 Dec 28;59(24):12815–20.

63. Yamakoshi J, Tokutake S, Kikuchi, M. Effect of proanthocyanidin-rich extract from grape seeds on human fecal flora and fecal odor. *Microb. Ecol. Health Dis*. 2001;13:25–31.

64. Tzounis X, Rodriguez-Mateos A, Vulevic J, Gibson GR, Kwik-Uribe C, Spencer JP. Prebiotic evaluation of cocoa-derived flavanols in healthy humans by using a randomized, controlled, double-blind, crossover intervention study. *Am J Clin Nutr*. 2011 Jan;93(1):62–72.

65. Jin JS, Touyama M, Hisada T, Benno Y. Effects of green tea consumption on human fecal microbiota with special reference to Bifidobacterium species. *Microbiol Immunol*. 2012 Nov;56(11): 729–39.

66. Carvalho-Wells AL, Helmolz K, Nodet C, Molzer C, Leonard C, McKevith B, Thielecke F, Jackson KG, Tuohy KM. Determination of the in vivo prebiotic potential of a maize-based whole grain breakfast cereal: a human feeding study. *Br J Nutr*. 2010 Nov;104(9):1353–6.

67. Costabile A, Klinder A, Fava F, Napolitano A, Fogliano V, Leonard C, Gibson GR, Tuohy KM. Whole-grain wheat breakfast cereal has a prebiotic effect on the human gut microbiota: a double-blind, placebo-controlled, crossover study. *Br J Nutr*. 2008 Jan;99(1):110–20.

68. Jarrett ME, Cain KC, Burr RL, Hertig VL, Rosen SN, Heitkemper MM. Comprehensive self-management for irritable bowel syndrome: randomized trial of in-person vs. combined in-person and telephone sessions. *Am J Gastroenterol*. 2009 Dec;104(12):3004–14.

69. Rubia K. The neurobiology of meditation and its clinical effectiveness in psychiatric disorders. *Biol Psychol*. 2009 Sep;82(1):1–11.

70. Chiesa A, Serretti A. A systematic review of neurobiological and clinical features of mindfulness meditations. *Psychol Med*. 2009 Nov 27:1–14.

71. Yao CK, Muir JG, Gibson PR. Review article: insights into colonic protein fermentation, its modulation and potential health implications. *Aliment Pharmacol. Ther*. 2016 Jan;43(2):181–96.

72. Reding KW, Cain KC, Jarrett ME, Eugenio MD, Heitkemper MM. Relationship between patterns of alcohol consumption and gastrointestinal symptoms among patients with irritable bowel syndrome. *Am J Gastroenterol.* 2013 Feb;108(2):270–6.

73. Abbasnezhad A, Amani R, Hajiani E, Alavinejad P, Cheraghian B, Ghadiri A. Effect of vitamin D on gastrointestinal symptoms and health-related quality of life in irritable bowel syndrome patients: a randomized double-blind clinical trial. *Neurogastroenterol Motil.* 2016 May 7. doi: 10.1111/nmo.12851.

INDEX

lactose intolerance 107–8
non-coeliac gluten sensitivity
105–6
possible causes 84–5
prebiotics for relief 176
probiotics for relief 172
questionnaire 20–2
remaining free of 198–204
understanding 23–5
see also daily diaries

T

temporomandibular joint disorder
33
10,000-step challenge 158
testing techniques
breath test 119–20, 135
coeliac disease 119
fructose intolerance 135
lactose intolerance 119–20
limitations of 37–8
melatonin levels 150–1
multiple problem foods 120
transit time, intestinal 25, 91
trauma, early childhood 137

V

vagus nerve 38, 46
vegetables
diet plan 187–90
FODMAP ratings 130
vegetarian enzymes 88
visceral hypersensitivity 38–9

W

water 194–5
wheat, food challenge 197
wholegrains 178

Y

yoga 158
yoghurt 174